IMPACT OF VISUAL SKILL ON MALE C...

By
G. SHIVAJI

DEDICATED
to
MY Beloved
FRIENDS

CONTENTS

CONTENTS

Chapter No.	Title	Page No.

CHAPTER - 1
INTRODUCTION

1.1	Nature of the game cricket	3
1.2	Visual Skills	5
1.2.1	Vision Training	10
1.2.2	Visual Skills	12
1.2.3	Importance of vision	12
1.2.4	Development of Vision	13
1.3	Vision and Motor Development	15
1.3.1	Vision and Sport Performance	16
1.3.2	Visual performance	19
1.3.3	Speed-Agility-and Visual Performance	19
1.3.4	The importance of Visual skills assessments	21
1.4	Visual Skill Variables	22
1.5	Skill Related Fitness Variables	24
1.6	Objective of this study	28
1.7	Statement of the problem	29
1.8	Hypotheses	29
1.9	Significance of the study	30
1.10	Delimitations	30
1.11	Limitations	31
1.12	Definition of the terms	31

Chapter No.	Title	Page No.
	CHAPTER - 2	
	REVIEW OF RELATED LITERATURE	
2.1	Studies on Visual Skills Fitness Training	33
	CHAPTER - 3	
	METHODOLOGY	
3.1	Selection of Subjects	53
3.2	Selection of Variables	53
3.3	Tools used in this study	54
3.4	Experimental Design	54
3.5	Reliability of Data	55
3.5.1	Instrument Reliability	55
3.5.2	Tester Competency	56
3.5.3	Orientation of Subjects	56
3.6	Pilot Study	56
3.7	Test Administration	56
3.8	Collection of Data – Pre-test	59
3.9	Administration of Training Programme	60
3.10	Training Procedure	60
3.10.1	Phase - I First four week Training Program	61
3.10.2	Phase - II Second four week Training Program	62
3.10.3	Phase - III Third four week Training Program	62
3.11	Description for Running Drills	63
3.11.1	Description for Visual Skill Drills	67
3.12	Collection of Data – Post - test	70
3.13	Statistical Technique	70

Chapter No.		Title	Page No.

CHAPTER - 4
ANALYSIS OF DATA AND RESULTS OF THE STUDY

4.1	Level of significance		71
4.2	Result of an Individualized Effect		71
4.3	Results of t - test		71
4.4	Results of Analysis of Variance		84
4.5	Results on Testing the Initials and Final Means		85
4.6	Results of Analysis of Covariance		86
4.7	Discussion on Findings		94

CHAPTER - 5
SUMMARY, CONCLUSIONS AND RECOMMENDATIONS

5.1	Summary		101
5.2	Findings		103
5.3	Conclusions		103
5.4	Recommendations		104

BIBLIOGRAPHY

LIST OF TABLES

LIST OF TABLES

Table No	Title	Page No
3.1	Tests Selection	54
3.2	Reliability Coefficients of Test Retest Scores of Criterion Variables	55
3.3	Phase - I First four week Training Program	61
3.4	Phase - II Second four week Training Program	62
3.5	Phase - III Third four week Training Program	63
4.1	Significance of mean gains / losses between pre and post test Visual Skill Fitness training Group (VSFTG) on selected visual skills and skill related fitness variables of male cricket players	72
4.2	Significance of mean gains / losses between pre and post test Control Group (CG) on selected visual skills and skill related fitness variables of male cricket players	78
4.3	Computation of Analysis of Variance of Initial Means of skill related fitness and visual skills variables	84
4.4	Computation of Analysis of Variance of Final Means of skill related fitness and visual skills variables	85
4.5	Computation of Analysis of Covariance of Adjusted post test means on Eye-hand co-ordination	86
4.6	Computation of Analysis of Covariance of Adjusted post test means on Visual Reaction Time	87
4.7	Computation of Analysis of Covariance of Adjusted post test means on Depth Perception	88
4.8	Computation of Analysis of Covariance of Adjusted post test means on Arm explosive power	89
4.9	Computation of Analysis of Covariance of Adjusted post test means on Leg explosive power	90
4.10	Computation of Analysis of Covariance of Adjusted post test means on Speed	91
4.11	Computation of Analysis of Covariance of Adjusted post test means on Agility	92
4.12	Computation of Analysis of Covariance of Adjusted post test means on Balance	93

LIST OF FIGURES

LIST OF FIGURES

Fig. No.	Title	Page No
4.1	Bar Diagram Showing the Mean Value of Pre-Test and Post-Test on Eye-hand co-ordination of VSFTG	74
4.2	Bar Diagram Showing the Mean Value of Pre-Test and Post-Test on Visual reaction time of VSFTG	74
4.3	Bar Diagram Showing the Mean Value of Pre-Test and Post-Test on Depth perception of VSFTG	75
4.4	Bar Diagram Showing the Mean Value of Pre-Test and Post-Test on Arm explosive power of VSETG	75
4.5	Bar Diagram Showing the Mean Value of Pre-Test and Post-Test on Leg explosive power of VSFTG	76
4.6	Bar Diagram Showing the Mean Value of Pre-Test and Post-Test on Speed of VSFTG	76
4.7	Bar Diagram Showing the Mean Value of Pre-Test and Post-Test on Agility of VSFTG	77
4.8	Bar Diagram Showing the Mean Value of Pre-Test and Post-Test on Balance of VSFTG	77
4.9	Bar Diagram Showing the Mean Value of Pre-Test and Post-Test on Eye-hand co-ordination of CG	80
4.10	Bar Diagram Showing the Mean Value of Pre-Test and Post-Test on Visual reaction time of CG	80
4.11	Bar Diagram Showing the Mean Value of Pre-Test and Post-Test on Depth perception of CG	81
4.12	Bar Diagram Showing the Mean Value of Pre-Test and Post-Test on Arm explosive power of CG	81
4.13	Bar Diagram Showing the Mean Value of Pre-Test and Post-Test on Leg explosive power of CG	82

Fig. No.	Title	Page No
4.14	Bar Diagram Showing the Mean Value of Pre-Test and Post-Test on Speed of CG	82
4.15	Bar Diagram Showing the Mean Value of Pre-Test and Post-Test on Agility of CG	83
4.16	Bar Diagram Showing the Mean Value of Pre-Test and Post-Test on Balance of CG	83
4.17	Adjusted Mean Values on Eye-hand co-ordination of VSFTG and CG	87
4.18	Adjusted Mean Values on Visual reaction time of VSFTG and CG	88
4.19	Adjusted Mean Values on Depth Perception of VSFTG and CG	89
4.20	Adjusted Mean Values on Arm explosive power of VSFTG and CG	90
4.21	Adjusted Mean Values on Leg explosive power of VSFTG and CG	91
4.22	Adjusted Mean Values on Speed of VSFTG and CG	92
4.23	Adjusted Mean Values on Agility of VSFTG and CG	93
4.24	Adjusted Mean Values on Balance of VSFTG and CG	94

CHAPTER I
INTRODUCTION

CHAPTER - I

INTRODUCTION

In sports success depends on player's ability to develop and perfect a specific set of perceptual, cognitive and motor skills. Visual skill fitness training is changing the sports world by using exercises that develop visual skills to improve performance, consistency, accuracy and stamina of the visual system. Visual skill fitness training and its needs has long been recognized by trainers and coaches in the game of coordinative abilities like cricket very long ago as the source for success of a player. Particularly in the game of cricket visual system plays a crucial role in guiding the player's search for essential information underlying skilful behavior.

Cricket is a game of coordinative abilities. In this game, player has to give importance to develop the coordinative abilities equivalent to physical aspects. Coordinative abilities are the product of body and mind. In the successful execution of players are in need of coordinative abilities like, reaction, coordination and perception. Coordinative abilities can be developed only sensory based physical training of visual skill training. Visual skills are the key to a cricket player's timing, co-ordination and overall performance. When the player trains, he most probably works on his aerobic capacity, endurance, strength, muscle tone and or flexibility. But, truth holds that he also needs to train his eyes. The stamina, flexibility and fine-tuning of the visual system can sometimes provide the split second timing the player needs to truly excel in cricket. Most players train every muscle in the body except the eye muscles.

Vision is both a learned and a developed skill. Of all the movement skills required in cricket, vision is the last skill to be fully developed to coordinate the movements related to ball handling and performing successfully in cricket. As the eyes lead, the body will follow, the eyes can be trained just like any other muscle in the body to improve reaction to what is seen. As such the role of physical exercise and practice in achieving the maximum results, the visual skills also can improve the performance of a player the game of cricket. Having this the present study was formed with the thirst of finding the changes on visual skills fitness variables when imparting the visual skill fitness training in addition to their physical training schedule in the game of cricket.

In sports success depends on player"s ability to develop and perfect a specific set of perceptual, cognitive and motor skills. In particular, the visual system plays a crucial role in guiding the player"s search for essential information underlying skilful behaviour. Visual skill fitness training is changing the sports world by using exercises that develop visual skills to improve performance, consistency, accuracy and stamina of the visual system.

Cricket is a game of coordinative abilities. In this game, player has to give importance to develop the coordinative abilities equivalent to physical aspects. Coordinative abilities are the product of body and mind. In the successful execution of players are in need of far as fundamental and advanced skills in cricket is concerned, coordinative abilities like, reaction, coordination and perception. Coordinative abilities can be developed only sensory based physical training of visual skill training. Visual skill fitness training and its needs has long been recognized by trainers and coaches in the game of coordinative abilities like cricket very long ago as the source for success of a player.

In the game of cricket effectiveness of the player"s ability to act quickly and accurately depends upon how efficient the visual system can process the information. Visual information is critical for performing a variety of motor skills that are used in cricket. When the players" movements must coincide with a changing environment, such as hitting the ball, catching the ball, or in motor activities requiring precise movements of the limbs in regards to a target.

When the players have better visual skills, they can make faster and better decisions. If the players have the time to make multiple decisions, they can more precisely implement those decisions and thus be more successful. According to Stahl (2001) vision, decision and anticipation can be improved during training sessions, playing smaller sized games in smaller areas. This will ensure that the players learn to think under pressure. This allows them to sharpen their decision making, anticipation and visual skills.

The eye is vital sensory receptor that supplies information regarding the movement of the objects in the environment. Visual search and attention are crucial components in the anticipatory decision making, response selection and execution the process. Earlier studies in this area evidenced significantly for progressive in nature, it"s developing the motor fitness components and psychomotor components of players. Those are needed for developing the performance of players.

Vision is one of the several sensory organs which receive information from the external environment and for years it has been recognized that many sports place demands on vision and particular visual skills.

1.1 Nature of the game cricket

The game is played on a large circular or oval shaped ground whose diameter is usually between 450-500 feet. Around the field there is either a rope or fence or a line drawn all around. This is known as the boundary. In the center of the field is the pitch where the actual battle between bat and ball takes place. At either end of this 22-yard pitch lines are drawn, behind which the stumps (3 upright rods) appear. The area between the line and the stumps is called the popping crease. The space between the stumps is so arranged that a cricket ball cannot pass through it. Two batsmen take the crease, the non-striker standing at the bowlers end and the other batsman called the striker who actually receives the ball when delivered by the bowler. When the batsmen are at the crease, the other players wait in the pavilion for their turn to come.

The batsmen wear helmets to protect themselves from deliveries which rise and also wear "pads" on both legs. They have guards to protect sensitive areas. They have bats which are straight on one side and humped on the other. The ball is made of hard cork and string ball covered with leather. The ball is red in color for a test match and white for a one-day match. They also wear gloves while batting. The wicketkeeper also wears gloves as he has to take hard catches and fielders fielding in close field positions also wear helmets. Leather shoes with spikes and long pants and shirts complete the outfit. The clothes are white if a test match is being played and colored if it is a one-day match. The batting side wears different colored clothes from the fielding side.

The ultimate object of the team that is batting first is to score as many runs as possible and the aim of the opponent would be to get all the batsmen out for as low a score as possible. To achieve this, the opposing team places its 10 fielders in vantage positions to restrict the scoring. The wicket keeper is always behind the batsman to gather any ball not played by him and also to hit the stumps with the ball in case the batsmen decide to take runs. If the batsmen cross over once from crease to crease, one run is scored. If the ball crosses the boundary a four is declared, and if it crosses the boundary without touching the ground, then a six is declared. The batsman is declared „bowled" if the ball hits the wicket (when the batsman fails to hit the ball), dislodging the bails placed on top of the stumps. If the batsman hits a ball and if it caught before it touches the ground, he is given out" caught", If he fails to regain his ground after hitting the ball and taking a run or runs, then he is declared " run out". If the ball hits the batsman on his leg in front of the wicket without hitting the bat and it is felt that it would have hit the stumps, he is declared out Leg Before Wicket , In attempting to play a shot, if the batsman is outside the popping crease and the wicketkeeper breaks the wicket, he is declare" stumped". If while attempting to hit the ball, the wicket is hit, he is given out "hit wicket". If after one batsman is out, the next batsman does not take the crease within the stipulated time, the batsman is declared out " timed out". The person who decides whether the batsman is out or not is called an "umpire". There are two umpires, one standing behind the stumps at the non-strikers end watching the bowler and the batsman carefully and another umpire to judge "run outs". The umpire raises his index finger if the batsman is declared "out". If the umpire is not sure, he can refer the decision to the "third umpire".

Two bowlers alternate the bowling attack bowling "over's" from opposite ends. Each over normally consists of 6 balls. If the bowler while delivering the ball has both feet beyond the crease, the ball is said to be a "no ball", and a run is given to the opposing team. If the ball is wide off the crease and the batsman is unable to play the ball, a wide is declared and the opposing team scores a run. Byes, leg byes, wides and no balls all constitute what is known as "extras". It is in the interest of the bowling team to restrict the number of extras. The umpire extends his arm horizontally and waves it forwards and backwards if it is a four, raises both arms above his head if it is a six, holds out an arm in a horizontal manner if it is a no ball and both arms extend horizontally if it is a wide.

When 10 players of a team are declared " out." the "innings" of that team comes to an end. The other team takes the field and tries to score more runs than its opponent. Depending on the nature of the game, there can be one innings (If it is a one day match) and two innings each if it is a test match. In the case of a one day match, the person scoring more runs is the winner, but in the case of a test match which lasts for 5 days, the match is said to be "drawn" if it is inconclusive and "tied" if both the teams score exactly the same number of runs.

1.2   Visual Skills

In recent years, there has been a growing acceptance that perceptual skills precedes and determines skilful actions in sport and other contexts (Harris &

Jenkin, 1998; Williams et al., 1999). In particular, the visual system plays a crucial role in guiding the player's search for essential information underlying skilful behaviour. One of the best explanations of what "visual search strategies" entails is that it can be said that visual search strategies refers to the way that the eyes move around the field in an attempt to direct visual attention towards relevant sources of information. According to Zelinsky et al. (1997) eye movement registration systems only provide information about the orientation of the fovea and, consequently, visual fixation may not always be indicative of information extraction. Many circumstances require the effective integration of information from the fovea, para-fovea and periphery (Williams & Davids, 1998).

Since almost 80% of the entire input that goes to the brain, comes from the eyes, it can be said that vision is one of the most important factors playing a role in sport (Hodge et al., 1999). The psychological and other aspects of sports performance like visual skills; psychology, nutrition, etc. are often neglected if not always. For a player to excel, attention should be given to all these aspects of skills enhancement (Hodge et al., 1999). Even mental toughness is a skill that can be trained and enhanced. At an elite level in cricket, there may be only five to fifteen percent difference between winning and losing, and this is where mental toughness accounts for that five to fifteen percent difference. Psychological skills develop through basic skill learning, fine-tuning and repetitive practice, which take determination and discipline (Hodge et al., 1999).

A sportsman's extraordinary performance depends on successfully using all of his or her available visual information. In recent years, there has been a growing acceptance that perceptual skill precedes and determined skilful actions in sport (Harris & Jenkin, 1998; Williams et al., 1999). The visual system plays a crucial role in guiding the player's search for essential information underlying skilful behaviour. When discussing visual search strategies, it is normally referred to as the way the eyes move around a display in an attempt to direct visual attention towards the relevant sources of information. According to Abernethy (1996) the role of vision can generally be accepted as a critical source of information for the planning and the executing of motor skills.

Visual performance in sport can be seen as an interaction between two visual systems. Abernethy (1986) introduced the visual system as a computer analogy of information gathering and processing by dividing the "analogy" into the two visual systems, namely the hardware and the software visual systems. The hardware visual system (skills) can be seen as the physical differences in the mechanical and the optometric properties of a person"s visual system and the software system (skills) can be seen as the cognitive differences in the analysis, selection, coding and general handling of the visual information during training and or competition. The hardware system consists of six optometric skills, being static and dynamic visual acuity, depth perception accommodation, fusion, colour vision, and contrast sensitivity (Abernethy, 1987).

There are seven optometric skills that form part of the software system, and they are eye hand co-ordination, eye-body co-ordination, visual adjustability, visual concentration, central-peripheral awareness, visual reaction time, and visualization (Ferreira, 2002). Accurate decision-making in sport depends largely on the level of attention, scanning for opportunities and then acting upon them, in a specific situation (Greenwood, 1993). The Visual skills necessary to conduct this accurate decision-making are the software skills.

The emphasis of coaching or training players in cricket has been heavily reliant upon repetition of motor skills, conditioning and weight training. Although strength and endurance are beneficial to the sport and can still be conducted without guidance by a coaching authority, repetition of motor skills is the key to any individual or team success and it should always be monitored to ensure that the skill is being repeated correctly. Kindal and Winkin (2000) stated that "practice makes permanent", which suggests that any action constantly repeated, whether correct or incorrect, will be engrained into an automatic response.

Competitive sports managers, coaches, athletes, and scientists have been searching for new ways to improve and to enhance sports performance to gain an advantage in their respective sports. Hopfinger et al. (2000) explained that dynamic interplay between the attentional control system and the sensory brain structures correlates to selective visual attention. Visual information is critical for performing a variety of motor skills that are used in cricket. This visual information is critical when the players" movements must coincide with a changing environment, such as hitting the ball, catching the ball, or in motor activities requiring precise movements of the limbs in regards to a target. The study of these movement activities, such as pointing at a target, relocating a body segment in space, or reaching for an object, has been directly linked to vision and movement control since the pioneering work of Woodworth in 1899 (Hopfinger et al., 2000). By "seeing with the mind"s eye," a cricket player is able to visualize the skill about to be performed.

According to Wilson and Falkel (2004) visualization can be taught, as can many other visual perceptual skills. These authors also argued that for athletes to perform at the highest level of competition, they have to be in tune with their visual motor and perceptual systems. Most players would never think about going into competition without having practiced their skills and improved their sport-specific strength and conditioning before the match (Wilson & Falkel, 2004). Visual skills fitness training exercises, like any other component of the player"s training regime, are necessary for optimal preparation for competition.

During the initial stages of performing a skill, players carry out visual search patterns to select from the playing environment certain clues that can be relevant for the performance demands of specific situations. Recent reviews have suggested that successful performance in sport requires skill in perception as well as efficient and accurate execution of movement patterns (Abernethy, 1987; Williams & Davids, 1994). When focusing on cricket, it is argued that the ability to quickly and accurately perceive events in complex sport settings is an essential requirement of skilled performance. For example, in cricket, the players are confronted with a rapidly changing, information-rich environment involving the cricket ball, other cricketers players (being either the opponents and or team mates), and the field of play. According to Bard and Fleury (1976) from a cognitive perspective, the cricket player has very little time in which to interpret all of the data available.

This is due to the player"s limited information processing capacity and the constrained circumstances due to the sport demands; therefore only the most pertinent information is selected and acted upon. McPherson (1994) stated that while there has been a limited examination of the development of perceptual and cognitive skills, such as anticipation and decision-making in sport, few, if any, studies have investigated the contribution of visual abilities to sporting expertise at different stages of development. It has long been apparent that the process of selecting relevant information, whilst disregarding less informative pieces of information is not conducted in an arbitrary manner. It is based on deliberate visual search strategies. These visual search strategies enable the skilled cricket player to make more efficient use of the time available for analysing of the skills. It has been argued that Visual skills fitness training exercises allow sportsmen and –women to improve their visual skills and thus improve their performance skills. Wilson and Falkel (2004) stated that the improvements from Visual skills fitness training exercises in eye movement skills, focusing skills, peripheral visual awareness, and visual perceptual skills will carry over onto the field of play. Thus helping the players to perform at their best and helping the players to reach the next level, no matter what level they are currently competing at.

1.2.1 Vision Training

Researchers have claimed that visual training can be the determining factor between winning and losing. Differences have been found between experts and novices on sport-specific pattern recognition and anticipation. It identified five visual skills for comparing professional to non- professional rugby players: eye-hand coordination, eye-body coordination, peripheral awareness, visual reaction time and visual concentration. Ninety-five (95) rugby players participated in this study. Although the professional players performed much better than the novice group, the authors concluded that there was room for improvement and they recommended that vision enhancement programmes be implemented for both groups. Another study compared the visual skills of ruby players from two different age groups (Venter & Ferreira, 2004). The older group outperformed the younger group on tests of the different visual skills. The authors speculated that the difference could have been due to a more advanced level of motor development or to more experience and coaching.

Leviton (1992) took the position that players and athletes need to exercise their eyes. He submitted that players can use eye exercises to enhance the ability of their eyes to relax, focus, shift, and work as a team, as well as to visualize. He stated that relaxation exercises are necessary to enhance blood circulation. Focusing exercises are necessary to strengthen the eyes" ability to quickly move from a near to a far point and then back again. Eye shifting exercises can discourage staring and help the eye to quickly move focus point from one visual field to another. Fusion exercises help to strengthen the ability of both eyes to work together in the same direction. Visualization develops memory, which leads to better recognition of objects and situations.

Leviton (1992) described a variety of possible visual skill training activities. He included activities such as bouncing on a trampoline while performing eye exercises. He suggested this would help the individual to learn to perform visually while at the same time improving general body coordination and improving the ability to pay attention. The inclusion of challenges to balance in sport vision training exercises was recommended because of the importance of postural control in sport. He was convinced that players should become aware of how movement, posture and alignment of their body can affect vision. Posture is the basis for head position. The more optimal the head position, the better view the eyes will have of the critical visual field.

The results for the expert group showed that their scan paths closely followed the presentation of important visual cues by the boxer on the screen, and that their visual search path was in the form of the circle. In the intermediate group the scan paths were also closely related to the presentation of visual cues, but this was not the case with the novices. The authors concluded that if training programmes are to help novices improve, they must include specific activities to help novices learn to identify cues and to control their visual search to attend to those cues in complex situations and when under pressure.

Success in meeting the challenges of a changing situation during game play relies on how well the player can integrate and interpret information and then develop and implement a plan for action (Knudson & Kluka, 1997). One important aspect of this process is the efficiency with which players use their eyes. Knudson and Kluka (1997) recommend vision training as one way in which the coach can help players learn to focus on certain visual cues. Different colour balls or markings on equipment can be valuable to draw a player"s attention and focus to certain visual cues.

Visual training exercises can be incorporated in training or even during the warm-up of the session. During these exercises, the different eye movements used during a particular sport can be practiced specifically. This special attention to visual skills development helps to coordinate different eye movements needed to get information from the environment. In fast-action sports, players must practice following fast-moving objects and move their body in response to the pressure of time and speed constraints.

1.2.2 Visual Skills

A wide range of visual skills that can be tested, but it is important to recognize which of these visual skills are important for the specific sport that is investigated. Planer (1994) previously published a sport vision testing battery and applied a 5-point performance scale for the different skills. In other words a superior group, above average group, average group, ineffective group and a needs immediate attention group. This was done according to the athletes" performances in the skills. Coffey and Reichow (1990) also proposed a visual skills testing battery, but did not divide the visual skills in the above categories. Buys (2002) used these two studies as a basis and developed norms for elite athletes based on the above 5-point categories. The rugby community has now realized the importance of vision in sport. Because of this realization, Ferreira (2001) submitted a testing battery of all the different visual skills that are important for rugby. Out of all these testing batteries it was decided to discuss the following visual skills.

1.2.3 Importance of vision

In cricket, vision is possible that success is achieved by accurately made decisions, based on the information obtained by visual input. Effectiveness of the player"s ability to act quickly and accurately depends upon how efficient the visual system can process the information. Efficient visual skills are one of the more important assets any player can have. When considering the favorite sport a sportsperson participates in, chances are that visual skills play a very important role in that specific activity (Wilson & Falkel, 2004). Accuracy, balance, concentration and co-ordination, are a few of the visually related abilities a player uses during sports event. Batting averages (e.g. in cricket), racquetball score; pass completion and free throw percentages can be affected by vision (www.drlampert.com, retrieved on 2004/02/05).

Vision involves many subtle and sophisticated links between the brain, muscles and eyes. During physical training a player works on the aerobic capacity, muscle endurance, muscle strength, muscle tone and/or flexibility (Wilson & Falkel, 2004). The stamina, flexibility and fine-tuning of the visual system can provide the player with the split-second timing needed to truly excel in the chosen sport. Vision has been found to be the most complex and the dominant sensory system used to provide feedback (Atkins, 1998). Good vision requires exceptional visual and/or perceptual skills, which involves the eyes feeding information to the brain. The brain then interprets the information and sets the arms, hands, legs, feet, and the body"s balance system in motion. It therefore instigates the appropriate physical action the player needs to play cricket. The late Blanton Collier (football coach) coined the phrase: "the eyes lead the body".

1.2.4 Development of Vision

According to Williams (1983) although the brain should not be considered a fixed entity in terms of learning, this might suggest that a sensitive period of development of sports related visual skills lies between birth and early teens. According to the author within this period of development, binocularity and depth perception appear to advance early on, improving between the ages of two and five years. According to Wikipedia (www.wikipedia.com, retrieved on 2007-08-01) "the normal human brain weighs between one and one-and-a half kilograms. An adult"s brain (also referred to as a matured human brain) consumes some 20 to 25% of the energy that is used by the body, while an infant"s brain (referred to as the developing brain) consumes around 60%".

Loran and MacEwen (1995) stated that vision is the ability to process or interpret the information, which is seen. It is postulated that vision training and visual skills were not considered to be that important in the everyday sport setting;

although athletes and trainers did do vision related training tests inadvertently (Loran & MacEwen, 1995).

These authors went on to explain that vision plays a big role in the athlete"s response times, eye-hand-body-coordination, balance, spatial orientation and anticipation. These activities should be examined not only in the laboratory, but also more in the exact environmental surroundings that those activities are performed in.

The visual system plays a crucial role in guiding the cricket and the soccer player"s search for essential information underlying skilful behaviour. When talking about visual search strategies, it refers to the way that the eyes move around a display in an attempt to direct the visual attention towards the relevant source of information. Sherman (1980) explained that when researchers investigate the "effect of the visual system on sport performance, one needs to understand the interplay between environmental demands on the visual system, optical properties of the eye, and the action capacity of the visual system".

From recent studies of motion perception in which continued figural changes of this type are presented without three-dimensional depth cues, overwhelming evidence indicates that the visual system spontaneously abstracts relational invariance in the optical flow and constructs precepts of rigid objects moving in three-dimensional space (Johansson, 1995). According to the author it has been found that continuous perspective transformations always evoke the perception of moving objects with a constant size and shape. The author explains that this means that the particular projection chosen perceptually by the visual system is one that represents Euclidean invariance under the conditions of motion in rigid three-dimensional space.

Each player"s visual system assists him in anticipating and responding more quickly to complex visual conditions. Clear vision and efficient visual skills are two of the more important assets a player can have. The cricket players" ability to act quickly and accurately is dependent upon how efficient the visual system can process the information of the task at hand. During a competitive game, the human body is pushed to perform on a higher level, both physically and mentally. According to Venter and Ferreira (2004) this places enormous stress "on the human body. As soon as this happens, the visual system might become obstructed".

According to Abernethy (1991a) motor development is the basis of skill acquisition. First there should be general gross motor development to form the basis for the fine motor development to take place; in other words the acquisition of motor and visual skills. By training cricket players to "utilize their visual search system, a coach can develop the capacity to detect the relevant information from the environment automatically" (Magill, 1998; Abernethy & Neal, 1999). "When this is achieved, it appears as the players are performing their tasks with ease, "Making a difficult task looks easy" (Magill, 1998; Abernethy & Neal, 1999).

1.3 Vision and Motor Development

Wilson and Falkel (2004) stated that when considering the favorite sport a sportsperson participates in, chances are that visual skills play a very important role in that specific activity. Co-ordination, concentration, balance and accuracy are just a few of the visually related abilities a player uses during any sports event. Vision can affect batting averages (e.g. cricket), racquetball score; pass completion and free throw percentages.

Eye-hand co-ordination skills can be defined as the ability to effectively respond to visual stimuli (O"Brian & Hayes, 1995). Williams and Grant (1999) explained that hand-eye co-ordination involves the integration of the eyes and the hands/body as a unit. Thus the eyes must lead and guide the motor system of the body (also known as the movement system). When a deficit is found in hand-eye co-ordination, it can be expected that the deficit can have an effect on all levels of performance that require movement of the player, bat, ball, etc. Since sport is typically performed under temporal constraints and varying levels of physiological stress or fatigue, attempts should be made to examine visual function under more realistic test conditions.

1.3.1 Vision and Sport Performance

In order to fully understand the contribution of vision to successful performance, a multifactorial approach to assessing skilled behaviour in sport is necessary (Ward & Williams, 2000). Helsen and Starkes (1999), together with Simonton (1999) investigated the amount of variance explained by a single factor that provides only limited insight into the complexity of sporting expertise and found that the literature for skill, and talent, are multidimensional in nature and consequently needs to be assessed using a multifactorial approach.

Visual skills are the key to a cricket player"s timing, co-ordination and overall performance. When the player trains, he most probably works on his aerobic capacity, endurance, strength, muscle tone and/or flexibility. But, truth holds that he also needs to train his eyes. The stamina, flexibility and fine-tuning of the visual system can sometimes provide the split second timing the player needs to truly excel in his specific sport (being it cricket or soccer). Most players train every muscle in the body except the eye muscles.

Vision is both a learned and a developed skill. Of all the movement skills required in cricket, vision is the last skill to be fully developed and the first to break down in performance. As the eyes lead, the body will follow. The eyes can be trained just like any other muscle in the body to improve reaction to what is seen. Just as exercise and practice increase strength and speed, so can the visual performance be improved to achieve maximum results.

Wilson and Falkel (2004) explained that vision involves two basic categories of function: visual motor and visual perceptual skills. These authors further stated that visual motor skill is probably the easiest category to relate to sport-specific performance. If a player can"t move his eyes quickly and effectively, then he cannot optimally perform sport specific tasks. It has been found that one of the primary differences between good and elite-level cricket players, other than their physical skills being equal, is that elite cricket players can move their eyes more effectively and efficiently for the duration of the game (Wilson & Falkel, 2004).

Motor skills development is very important because the movement of different body parts must be co-ordinate to produce a total movement (Davis et al., 1995). These motor skills will become better and more controlled as the child matures and gets stronger. Davis et al. (1995) pointed out that it is also very important because these motor skills are used in sports performances. There are three basic ocular motor skills used in the visual motor system, namely vergence, focusing, and tracking. Wilson and Falkel (2004) stated that it is important for the eyes to be able to converge (or cross) as the ball comes towards the player or diverge (or uncross) as the ball goes away. It is also necessary for the player to be able to focus on the target where he wants to place the ball (either with the bat, or with his foot as to where to kick the ball) and then to be able to track the specific target smoothly through space (Wilson & Falkel, 2004).

Tracking is the ability of the eyes to follow an object, in this study the cricket ball, from one point to another. The first movement category is Pursuit eye movement; this is the ability of the eyes to smoothly follow the ball through space (Wilson & Falkel, 2004). The second movement category is Saccadic eye movement, which is the quick jumping movement of the eyes from one point to another. Pursuits and Saccades are often used in sports and everyday life to perform both simple and complex tasks (Wilson & Falkel, 2004).

Successful performance in sport requires skill in perception as well as the efficient and accurate execution of the movement patterns. According to Williams et al. (1999) the awareness that skilled perception preceded appropriate action has led researchers to examine the role it plays in sport performance. A player's ability to use advance postural clues is particularly important in fast ball sports, such as soccer and cricket, where the speed of play, the drastically changing angles, and the ball's velocity dictate such decisions. These must often be made in advance of the action.

Researchers have typically relied on verbal reports or event occlusion techniques and a few attempts have been made to record goalkeepers' visual behaviour using eye movement registration techniques (Williams et al., 1999). Most of those involved in eye movement research in sport have attempted to identify differences in visual behaviour as a function of age, skill or experience.

According to Williams and Davids (1997) visual concentration is not only dependent on good visual abilities. There are other factors that also contribute to optimal visual performance, e.g. confidence, the amount of practice the player puts in and being aware of the situation that he is in. Attentional selectivity and the ability to perform two or more skills concurrently play an important role in sports performance (Williams & Davids, 1997).

Williams et al. (1999) stated that "skilled performers do not necessarily possess superior visual hardware compared with their less skilled counterparts". Experts demonstrated superior skills in recognizing, recalling and semantically classifying visual information. The hardware visual system should be developed to an average level of performance to eliminate any potential limits on the software visual skills (Williams et al., 1999).

From a sports science point of view, one can see that cricket are games where the players and the ball are almost constantly in motion, with the ball changing direction at acute angles very often. Soccer is a game where there is no "time out" to call all the players together or the ability to stop play by catching and throwing the ball (except the goal keeper). It is postulated that over 90% of the time, a cricket player uses his vision to put all of these skills into action (Morris, 2000).

Research has proven that visual motor skills can be improved through Visual skills fitness training to allow for optimal visual motor performance during sports. The visual system actually performs much better after it has been loaded, or stressed (Wilson & Falkel, 2004). The goal of Visual skills fitness training programmes is to improve ocular motor skills and to enhance not only visual performance but also sports performance. Wilson and Falkel (2004) argued that when you improve the ocular motor skills (vergence, focusing, and tracking) you improve athletic performance.

1.3.2 Visual performance

Visual performance in sport is an interaction between two visual systems. Abernethy (1986) introduced the visual system as a computer analogy of information gathering and processing and dividing the "analogy" into the two visual systems, being the hardware and the software visual systems. According to the author the hardware system (skills) can be seen as the physical differences in the mechanical and the optometric properties of a person"s visual system and the software system (skills) can be seen as the cognitive differences in the analysis, the selection, coding and general handling of the visual information during training or competition. Ferreira (2002) explained that the hardware system consists of six optometric skills, being static and dynamic visual acuity, depth perception, accommodation, fusion, color vision, and contrast sensitivity.

1.3.3 Speed-Agility-and Visual Performance

All aspects of cricket training and preparation are designed to maximize ability. Regardless of whether or not a cricket player has been genetically gifted with strong speed and agility traits, a player can dramatically improve his speed and agility by treating quick movements as a skill and training as such. Fitness is often thought of in terms of strength, endurance, flexibility and body conditioning. According to Barnes and Attaway (1996), cited in Roper (1998) agility has been defined as the ability of the player to change direction quickly and easily. Some objectives of agility training are enhanced power, balance, speed, and co-ordination (Barnes & Attaway, 1996).

Motor skills, which bridges the gap between fitness and technical ability is vital in training for cricket excellence. The body must be trained to respond to what the eyes sees. The eyes cannot be trained in isolation, the body must be taught to work as a unit. The long hours most cricket players spend in the gym and on the field working to improve their physical ability are important, however, they also need to concentrate on their visual skills.

Pearson (2004) speed, agility, quickness and multi-directional explosion are key components of the physical demands required of a cricket player. All aspects of cricket, including fielding, bowling, batting and wicket keeping, require the ability to move with speed, power and precision. The author stated that since the cricket revolution of the late seventies and early eighties, the game of cricket at all levels has evolved into a dynamic contest. Many aspects of the game are about the ability of the players to rapidly decelerate, redirect and accelerate as well achieving high speed.

These superb acts of speed, agility and quickness make the difference between winning and losing at whatever level of the game is played (Pearson, 2004). Cricket and soccer is a very athletic game, and therefore it is crucial that speed, agility and explosive acceleration are trained for and practiced. Speed, agility and visual training should be an adjunct to the overall conditioning and training of the cricket player"s training programme. By including the Visual skills fitness training programme in each training session (whether training on his own or with the team), the player and the coach will find that the player can perform better because he can "see" what he should have "been seeing" all the time.

According to Pearson (2004), a crucial part of any player"s game is the ability to cover the ground efficiently and economically over the first few meters and then to open up stride length and increase stride frequency when working over

40 to 50 meters. The author postulated that training to improve maximum speed requires a great deal of focus on correct running mechanics, stride length and frequency, the leg cycle and hip height or hip length. Pearson (2004) made it clear that focusing on the mechanics of running helps to control and use this power efficiently and sparingly. Training when fresh is also crucial for a player to attain maximum speed.

1.3.4 The importance of Visual skills assessments (Sports Vision testing)

The aim of sports vision is to train the player"s visual co-ordination and to gain knowledge of the motor response, which is what the eyes tell the body to do or better how to react to a specific visual stimulus. Williams and Horn (1995) pointed out that the average sports person has certain visual skills that are not that much different from the general public. Peripheral awareness enables the player to be aware of what is happening in his surrounding environment without actually looking at it (Williams et al., 1999).

It has been found that in sport (especially team sports), there is a lot of information that needs to be processed, e.g. the player has to be aware as to where the other players (team mates and opponents) are, has to watch the ball all the time and the player has to be able to anticipate where the next move is going to come from (Williams & Davids, 1994; Williams & Davids, 1997; Magill, 1993).

According to Knudson and Kluka (1997) "visual abilities affects sport performance, the acquisition of motor skills and can be improved by training". From the literature quoted thus far in this study, it is safe to postulate that there is no single area of sports performance where vision does not play a major role – throwing, catching, hitting, kicking, and judging field position, an opponent"s speed, team action and many more. Yet studies show that more than 30% of all players, including professionals, suffer from vision deficiencies that affect their sports performance to some degree. Non-athletes, as a group, have an even higher rate of vision problems and may explain why they are not participating in sport in the first place (Knudson & Kluka, 1997).

1.4 Visual Skill Variables

1.4.1 Eye-hand coordination

Eye –hand coordination is the ability involves the integration of the eyes and hands to function as a unit. The eyes must guide the body to execute the correct motor response. It is a perceptual- motor skill that involves the integration and processing of visual information in the central nervous system so that purposeful motor movements can be made (Abernethy, 1987). It can be a measure of the ability of an athlete to accurately and quickly respond to a stimulus (Ferreira, 2001). This is not just about the skill, but how fast the athlete can complete the movement.

This ability is due to the integration and processing in the central nervous system of visual information so that he/she can execute a perfect and precise movement (Sherman, 1980). It can be pro-active where a rugby player for instance reacts to pass a ball or re-active, where his team mate reacts to catching the ball. When an athlete constantly makes a wrong move, this skill needs improvement (Ferreira, 2001). The eyes determine what is going on (perception), the brain decides what to do (decision making) and the body then reacts on it (response) (Ferreira, 2001, Loran, MacEwen, 1995).

According to Elmurr (2000), athletes" eye-hand coordination on the Acuvision 1000 is 20% quicker than your non-athletic group. This ability can be evaluated by using a Saccadic fixator device. The athletes are instructed to press the button next to the red light. The light then moves randomly to another light on board and will go off as soon as athletes press the light. In rugby, motor responses are controlled by time and space; therefore this skill is very critical for the game of rugby(Ferreira, 2001).

1.4.2 Visual Reaction Time

Visual reaction time is the ability to perform the skills are very important. However, the time it takes the athlete to execute the movements is just as important. Thus, visual reaction time is the time the athlete receives information from the environment and decides to act on it in a certain way (Abernethy, 1991). The time and accuracy of the movement distinguishes the exceptional athlete from the novice. It is very similar to the eye-hand coordination skill, but with visual reaction time, the pro-action and the re-action parts are combined.

In a study done by Christenson and Winkelstein (1988) they concentrated on visual reaction time or motor reaction time as they called it. The test was done by instructing the athlete to use only his/her preferred hand. There is some sense in this as the hand they prefer is mostly the dominant one, but it also should be considered in context to the sport that is under investigation.

1.4.3 Depth Perception

Depth Perception is usually distinguished from other processes involving thought consciousness and judgment. According to Bartley (1958) perception is a form of discriminating behavior which involves an overall activity of a person immediately following or accompanying the stimulation of the sense organs. Perception is knowledge through the senses of existence and properties of matter and the external world. It causes actions which in turn change it and it is a continuous process. Friedman et al (1961) offers a clear distinction between sensation and perception that helps us to understand these terms better. A sensation involves "the presence of apparatus and means for reception of stimuli". Perception, on the other hand, involves "the presence of apparatus and means for the interpretation of stimuli".

The role of perception in motor learning and performance is a positive one evident. A person"s ability to receive and distinguish among available cues in a given situation enables him to perform more skillfully. There is no doubt that the senses underlie perception and that several senses probably interact simultaneously during the perceptive process. While spiking, the volleyball player concentrates on the ball and disregards irrelevant uses. Similarly, in the successful blocking, player requires attention to the feel of the ball movement and concentration on the direction and point of application of force that he has applied (Singer, 1968).

Perception depends on differences between stimuli and perceptibility or ease of discrimination, In volleyball, a player has to concentrate and attend at once to be successful in exacting his solves in high level stressful situations; otherwise his performance will be hampered. Perception is also influenced by factors namely personality, attitudes, emotional factors, experience and expectations, in addition to environmental variables.

1.5 Skill Related Fitness Variables

1.5.1 Muscular Power

Muscular power is the ability to release maximum force as fast as possible. It is a maximum muscular contraction against a resistance in a minimum amount of time. Power is a product of force and velocity. It is a compound element of motor fitness. It needs specific muscular strength, speed of limb movement and skill in integrating and co-coordinating the action. Increased velocity of parts of the body is related to improved neuromuscular initiation, co-ordination and precision of movement patterns. When a highly skilled level is attained, further performance improvement is primarily attributable to the increase in strength. Muscular power exists in its own right. Strength and power are separate entities.

Successful sporting performance at elite levels of competition often depends heavily on the explosive leg power of the athletes involved. Many team sports also require high levels of explosive power, such as Basketball, Volleyball,

Netball and the Rugby and Football codes for success at elite levels of competition. Explosive power comes from the development of speed strength and pure strength. Power represents the amount of work a muscle or muscle group can produce per unit of time. Until recent years power as it relates to sports performance has been the subject of limited research, but in the last decade or so researchers has realized the importance of training for power in a wide variety of sporting activities (Clutch et al, 1983).

Vertical and horizontal jumping, in its many different forms, requires high levels of explosive muscular power. Note power as the equivalent of explosive strength. Power is the equivalent of explosive strength. The term "speed-strength" synonymous with power. Paavolaienen et al (1999) suggested that muscle power is the ability of neuromuscular system to produce power during maximal exercise when glycolytic and oxidative energy production is high and muscle contractility may be limited.

1.5.1.1 Explosive Power

Successful sporting performance at elite levels of competition often depends heavily on the explosive leg power of the athletes involved. Vertical and horizontal jumping, in its many different forms, requires high levels of explosive muscular power. Power is the equivalent of explosive strength. "Speed-strength" is synonymous with power. Team sports such as hockey, volley ball, netball, rugby and football require high level of explosive power for success at elite levels of competitions. Explosive power comes from the development of speed and strength. (Paavolaienen et.al. 1999) suggested that muscle power is the ability of neuromuscular system to produce power during maximal exercise when glycoltics and oxidative energy production is high and muscle contractility may be limited. According to (Matavulj, 2001) the strength of the muscles in the limbs is moving and supporting the weight of the body repeatedly over a given period of time. In terms of dynamics strength, sometimes it has been called velocity or speed.

1.5.1.2 Leg Explosive Power

The strength of the muscles in the limbs is moving and supporting the weight of the body repeatedly over a given period of time in terms as dynamics strength, sometimes, it has been called velocity or speed. The important aspect of this factor is the requirement that the muscular force must be repeated as many times as possible. Explosive strength and dynamic strength involve movement of the body or of its limbs.

1.5.2 Speed

Speed is the ability to move the body or a part of the body as rapidly as possible from one point to another. It is the rate of movement, or the amount of time it takes for a body or object to travel between two points. Speed is obviously extremely important in all forms of racing, but also in team and goal related sports when someone has the chance to 'runaway' from the opposition. One of the major requirements in many sports is speed. In sports such as sprinting, soccer, cycling, hockey, fencing, games and many other team sports, speed is a major factor determining the overall outcome. In fact, all skill-related components contribute to speed. Speed requires the expenditure of a large amount of energy in a short period. . It is an important factor in almost all court and field games. It can make the difference in whether a performer is able to gain an advantage over his opponent. In games like basketball, football, hockey, and team hand ball both acceleration speed and running speed are basic to success (Jensen and Fisher, 1979).

Performing sports skills economically with ease, correct positioning of body levers and good neuro-muscular coordination will result in efficient use of energy and a higher speed of the movement. In addition to relaxation ability, joint flexibility is an important ingredient for performing movements with high amplitude (e.g. long stride in running) which in many sports is essential to execute optimum range of movement for maximum speed. Speed is determined not only by mobility and well synchronized neuro-muscular response but also by the frequency of the precise nervous impulses and strong concentration. This is because quick, explosive movements depend on a high level of power. Willpower and strong concentration are very important factors in achieving high speed. Exercises of will must be included in the training process to achieve a high level of speed.

Fast movements are performed by recruiting the fast twitch fibres, and because of their function and metabolic qualities these fibers constitute the most favorable preconditions for speed performances; for instance, successful sprinters have more than 60 percent fast twitch fibers, as a result of their genetic aptitude. Whereas has stated that speed is the result of both positive and negative forces. Muscular contractions are positive forces, while air or water resistance, gravity, friction, and inertia are some examples of negative forces. Increases in speed can result from decreasing the influence of the negative forces, or both. This illustrates the importance of individualizing training on the basis of the sport or event (Devries, 1974).

1.5.3 Agility

Agility is important in all activities that require quick changes in positions of the body and its parts. In hockey, fast starts and stops and quick changes in direction are fundamental to good performance. Agility enables an individual to rapidly and precisely alter the position and direction of the body and is an important ingredient for successful participation in a wide variety of sports. An agile person can quickly and efficiently mobilize the large muscle groups of the body in order to make rapid changes in direction of movement. Agility involves coordinating quickly and accurately the big muscles of the body in a particular activity. One's level of agility is probably a result of both innate capacity and training and experience. It is revealed to a great extent in sports involving efficient footwork and quick changes in body position force (Barrow and McGee, 1979).

1.5.4 Balance

Balance is an ability to maintain the center of gravity of a body within the base of support with minimal postural sway. When exercising the ability to balance, one is said to be balancing. Balancing requires concurrent processing of inputs from multiple senses, including equilibrioception (from the vestibular system), vision, and perception of pressure and proprioception (from the somatosensory system), while the motor system simultaneously controls muscle actions. The senses must detect changes of body position with respect to the base, regardless of whether the body moves or the base moves.

Age-related decline in the ability of the above systems to receive and integrate sensory information contributes to poor balance in older adults (Schmitz, 2007). As a result, the elderly are at an increased risk of falls. In fact, one in three adults aged 65 and over will fall each year. In the case of an individual standing quietly upright, the limit of stability is defined as the amount of postural sway at which balance is lost and corrective action is required. The limit of stability may be described by an irregular conical envelope above the support base (Hutchinson & Karen, 1995).

Lubetzki-Vilnai & Kartin, (2010) Balance can be severely affected in individuals with neurological conditions. Patients who suffer a stroke or a spinal cord injury for example, can struggle with this ability. It has also been determined that impaired balance is strongly associated with future function and recovery in some cases, particularly in stroke patients. Additionally, balance problems have been identified as the strongest predictor of falls.

1.6   Objective of this study
The objectives of this study are as follows:
1. To identify the status of visual skills (eye-hand coordination, visual reaction time and depth perception) and skill related fitness variables (arm explosive power, leg explosive power speed, agility and balance) of male cricket players at inter collegiate level.

2. To determine the effect of visual skills fitness training programe on selected visual skills and skill related fitness variables of male cricket players.

3. To study the comparative effects between the visual skill fitness training and control group (conventional training group) on selected visual skills and skill related fitness variables of male cricket players.

1.7 Statement of the problem

Now a day sport is being a highly competitive and commercialized one. Everybody in sport now recognize the increasing and essential need of visual and mental abilities rather than only train the physical abilities and skills to achieve the edge over the competitors. Visual skills training exercises are necessary for optimal preparation for competition. As a method of performance enhancement, it has been proven one in bringing the players to perform well at all levels of competition. Thus in the present scenario, research on visual skills and its impact on players performance in the game of cricket, requires as a need of hour. With this specific purpose, the present study was designed to find out the effect of visual skill fitness training programme on selected visual skills and skill related fitness variables of male cricket players

1.8 Hypotheses

The hypotheses formulated in the present study were as follows.

1. In studying the individualized effect, it was hypothesized that visual skill fitness training would significantly develop the visual skills and skill related fitness variables of male cricket players from the base line to post treatment.

2. It was further hypothesized that visual skill training may have significant improvements in developing the visual skills and skill related fitness variables of male cricket players than the conventional training group.

1.9 Significance of the study

The present study would have significant impact in the following aspects.

1. Results identified on status of visual skills and skill performance variables helping the players to identify their level of performance on selected visual skills and skill related fitness variables. It enables the physical education teachers and coaches to understand the importance of visual skill fitness training towards development of skill in sports. By imparting the visual skills as a part of the regular training schedule to performance of visual skills and skill related fitness variables can be improved.

2. Physical education teacher and coaches can certainly be benefited to manage their players especially during the period of competitive situation by availing the data on selected visual skills and skill related fitness variables. The visual skills can be used as treatment to have the positive changes on the performance of visual skills and skill related fitness of cricket players is a compatible one as compared to other training.

1.10 Delimitations

The study was delimited in the following aspects:

1. Subjects of the present study were delimited to 30 cricket players who were the participants of inter-collegiate level tournament.

2. As visual skills it was delimited to eye-hand co-ordination, visual reaction time and depth perception.

3. As skill related fitness components it was delimited to arm explosive power. Leg explosive power, speed, agility and balance.

4. The player's age ranged from 19 to 24 years.

5. The period of training programme was delimited to 12 weeks.

1.11 Limitations

The following factors are considered as limitations in the present study.

1. The life style, food habits and the family background of the subjects are to be considered as limiting factors.

2. The influence of individual motivational structure on the response of data is not taken into account.

3. The influence of socio economic conditions prevailing in the performance of criteria variables are also considered as a limiting factor.

4. The basic of knowledge of the subjects in exercise science and their previous experience of physical activities were not taken into consideration.

5. Since the subjects were motivated verbally during testing and training periods no attempt was made to differentiate their level of motivation.

6. The heredity factors of the subjects and their influence on the selected variables were not taken into consideration.

1.12 Definition of the terms

Visual skills

Visual skill is a capacity to accurately read the optic array. Visual skills therefore include a cognitive element. In other words, factors such as past experience will influence the ability to interpret the visual information. A visual ability involves the reception of visual information while a visual skill involves the perception of visual information. It is important to note that visual abilities support visual skills (Bressan, 2000).

Eye-hand coordination

Eye-hand coordination involves the integration of the eyes and the hands. It determines the effectiveness of a perceptual motor response to a visual sensory stimulus (Buys, 2002 & Ferreira, 2001).

Visual reaction time

Visual reaction time is the time required to perceive and respond to visual stimulation (Buys, 2002 & Ferreira, 2001).

Depth Perception

Depth perception is the ability to see the world in three dimensions and to perceive distance. Although this ability may seem simple, depth perception is remarkable when you consider that the image projected on each retina is two-dimensional. From these flat images, we construct a vivid three-dimensional world. To perceive depth, we depend on two main sources of information: binocular disparity, a depth cue that requires both eyes; and monocular cues, which allow us to perceive depth with just one eye.

Explosive Power

It is the capacity of the individual to release maximum force in a short period of time.

Speed

Speed is the capacity of the individual to perform successive movements of the same pattern at a faster rate.

Agility

Ability of the body or parts of the body to change direction rapidly and accurately.

Balance

Balance is an ability to maintain the center of gravity of a body within the base of support with minimal postural lean.

CHAPTER II
REVIEW OF RELATED LITERATURE

CHAPTER – II

REVIEW OF RELATED LITERATURE

2.1 Studies on Visual Skills Fitness Training

Literature survey comprises locating, reading and evaluating reports of research as well as reports of casual observation and opinion that are related to the individuals planned as research report. A study of relevant literature is an essential step to get a full picture of what has been done with regard to the problem under study. The investigator has made an attempt to bring a brief review of research related to the present study to form the background for the present study and presented the same with appropriate headings. In this section the studies related to effects of visual skills fitness training variables related to the present study are presented.

Studies on Vision Training

Joanne and Abernethy (1997) investigated that sports vision training programs can enhance visual skills and the level of sporting performance. Thirty young subjects were assigned equally to visual training, reading (placebo), and control groups. Visual and motor tests were administered before and after 4 weeks of training or control activity to determine whether any improvements in performance had occurred. Significant improvements on some aspects of vision were apparent for the visual training group, but their improvements in both vision and motor performance were no greater than for either of the other groups. There was no evidence for visual training improving either visual or motor performance beyond levels due simply to test familiarity. The benefits of the visual training exercises commonly used by optometrists to enhance sports performance are therefore open to question.

Paul et al., (2011) evaluated the effects of sports vision and eye hand coordination training on sensory and motor performance of table tennis players. 45 University level table tennis players were randomly divided into 3 equal groups of n=15. The experimental group underwent 8 weeks of sports vision and eye hand co-ordination training. The placebo group read articles pertaining to sports performance and watched televised table tennis matches, while the control group followed only routine practice sessions for 8 weeks. Measures of visual function and motor performance were obtained from all participants before and immediately after 8 weeks of training. Statistically significant pre to post training differences were evident by better improvement in visual variables and motor performance for the experimental group as compared to placebo and control. The present study therefore concluded that visual training program improves the basic visual skills, which in turn are transferable into sports specific performance.

Balasaheb et al., (2008) to investigate the influence of specific visual training program on batting performance in cricket players. Thirty club level male cricket batsmen were randomly divided into three equal groups. The experimental group followed six weeks of visual training program, on alternate days. The placebo group was given simple reading material and watched televised cricket matches for six weeks' duration, while the control group followed routine cricket practice. Pre- and post- test results were obtained for reaction time, depth perception, accommodation, saccadic eye movements and batting performance. Statistical analysis indicated significant improvement in all mentioned visual variables and batting performance in the experimental group ($p<0.001$). The placebo ($p<0.05$) and control group ($p<0.05$) also showed some improvement in batting performance but no significant improvement in visual variables was observed ($p>0.05$). It can be concluded that the visual training program improves visual skills of cricketers, which could lead to improvement in the batting performance.

Kruger et al., (2009) to determine the role and the impact of a visual skills training programme on the skills performance of cricket players, and whether visual training programmes are beneficial to competitive sports performance. Highly skilled cricket players (n=13) who were actively participating at a provincial level of competition, served as participants. Since the sample was relatively small non-parametric statistics, i.e. Wilcoxon test was used to analyze data. After initial testing the cricket players participated in an eight-week visual skill and performance skills programme for 60 minutes a day, once a week. The programme included sports vision activities, speed and agility activities and ball skills activities. The pre-training and post-training values of the cricket players were recorded and significance of difference was determined by using the Wilcoxon signed-ranks test. Data revealed that the visual skills programme had a significant influence on most of the tested variables (ball handling skills, co-ordination, visual awareness, eye tracking skills, accuracy, peripheral awareness, pro-action – reaction skills and visual concentration). It can thus be concluded that there was an increase in most of the variables tested (ball handling skills, co-ordination, visual awareness, eye tracking skills, accuracy, peripheral awareness, pro-action – reaction skills and visual concentration). Visual skills training, utilizing the conditions in this investigation can result in an increase in the players" visual fields. Visual skills training programmes can be beneficial to competitive sports performance.

Ludeke and Ferreira (2003) to evaluate the difference in the visual skill level of professional versus non-professional rugby players. The software visual skills, involving skills such as eye hand coordination, eye-body coordination, central- peripheral awareness, and reaction time, were examined. The results indicate that the professional players did outperform the nonprofessional players on all these skills except for visual concentration. Not all the results were however statistically significant. The importance of the above skills in the game of rugby is discussed and recommendations as to the implementation of vision enhancement programmes are made.

Toit et al., (2011) to determine if sports vision exercises could improve visual skills and there enhance motor and cognitive performance. A 169 second year physiology students (18-22 years of age) participated in the study. The students were divided into two control (n=78) and experimental groups (n=91) and pre and post sports vision tests were conducted. This included testing visual skill such as visual acuity, eye dominance, focusing, tracking, vergence, sequence, eye-hand co-ordination, visualization and reflex. The results showed a significant improvement in the sequencing and eye-hand coordination test in the experimental group. Whilst a non-significant improvement (control group) was observed in the visual acuity, visualization, tracking, vergence and reflex tests. The improvements (expert for focusing) were greater in the experimental group than in the control group. The study clearly showed that correct sports vision training can improve certain visual skills and lead to an enhancement of motor and cognitive learning and performance. Sports vision exercises are therefore an efficient method of improving certain visual skills and possibly minimizing any defects caused by stress.

Lluïsa Quevedo et al., (1999) Fencing sports required Motility, hand-eye reaction time, Dynamic visual acuity. The limitation programme was to Tasks , Postures , Working distances ,Visual acuity , Dynamic visual acuity , Binocular vision , Depth perception , Peripheral vision , Colour vision , Additional factors , Sunshine and artificial lighting , Hazards 20 male and 20 female students in physical education aged 18 to 21 yr. were each randomly assigned to both the experimental and control groups. Experimental subjects were given the 8-wk. Group differences were examined by using T tests Statistical analysis indicated significant gains in the four mentioned variables for the experimental group. The control group also showed significant differences in the visual variables but no significant improvement in static balance. Fencing performance was observed between groups. This study therefore provided evidence that a visual training awareness programme can improve sport performance in a visually demanding sport.

Potgieter and Ferreira (2009) to identify the visual skills important to rhythmic gymnasts and to explore whether these skills could be improved by means of an intervention programme. This study further aims to provide sport specific visual performance standards to the gymnasts. Little research is available connecting vision to this sport and it was seen as a good opportunity to make a difference. After testing the visual skills of a sample of 62 rhythmic gymnasts (divided randomly into two comparable groups of 32 for the experimental group and 30 for control group) the experimental group followed a sports specific intervention programme while the control group adhered to their regular training schedule. The visual skills trained by the intervention programme were re-tested on both the experimental and control groups of gymnasts. The results obtained from the post-intervention measurements were analyzed and compared to the original data obtained from the pre-intervention measurements of both the groups of gymnasts. Results from competitions were obtained and compared to establish the effect of the intervention programme. It is concluded that the software skills of the visual system plays an important role in the sport of rhythmic gymnastics. These skills can be improved by implementing a sustainable visual training programme for the training of rhythmic gymnasts.

Bressan (2003) to determine the effectiveness of three different approaches to improving sports performance through improvements in "sports vision:" (1) a visual skills training programme, (2) traditional vision coaching sessions, and (3) a multi-disciplinary approach identified as sports vision dynamics. Seventy women (ages of 19-24) were matched on the basis of their netball passing skills and their performance on visual skills tests, in order to form four groups of similar abilities. The intervention programmes were conducted in 30-minute sessions, twice a week for five consecutive weeks. Group 1 received vision dynamics; Group 2 received vision coaching; Group 3 received visual skills training; and Group 4 was the control group. All three groups receiving vision enhancement interventions achieved a significant increase in their netball passing speed. Subjects receiving vision dynamics and visual skills training also achieved a significant increase in their passing accuracy. The percentage of improvement in both speed and accuracy gains indicated that the vision dynamics programme produced much greater gains than either of the other two treatment programmes. These results indicate that sports vision dynamics appear to be the most effective approach to helping players maximise their use of vision during sport performance.

Strydom and Ferreira (2010) to determine the most important visual skills applicable to archery and secondly to determine the norms for these visual skills necessary for an archer to perform at an elite level. Another goal was to compare our results with previous results for elite athletes, (determined by Buys in 2002). Twenty eight archers from different archery styles such as compound bow archery, resurvey bow archery and traditional bow archery were used. Their visual skill norms were categorized as Superior, above average, Average, Ineffective and Needs immediate attention. The results indicated that visual acuity, contrast sensitivity, stereopsis, eye-hand coordination, eye body coordination and visual response time may be the most important skills in archery. Other factors such as distance judging and the choice of monocular or binocular aiming has also been tested and discussed and norms for these tests were also established.

Spaniol et al., (2011) to investigate the relationship between visual skills and tennis performance of NCAA Division I tennis players. Visual skills were assessed by the Visual Edge® Performance Trainer (VEPT), a commercial software program designed to evaluate eye alignment, depth perception, convergence, divergence, visual recognition, and visual tracking. Tennis performance was determined by team player ranking (TPR). Eleven NCAA Division I tennis players (6 males, mean ± SD, age = 20.8 ± 1.3 yr, height = 181.6 ± 8.2 cm, weight

74.9 ± 5.2 kg; 5 females, age = 20.6 ± 1.3 yr, height 169.3 ± 4.2 cm, weight = 65.0 ± 10.7 kg) participated in the study. A non-significant t-test indicated that visual skills are not gender specific, and therefore males and females could be evaluated as one group. The results showed significant correlations between final VEPT scores and TPR ($r = -0.61$; $p = 0.046$), final VEPT score rank and TPR ($r = 0.54$; $p = 0.089$), visual tracking percent correct and TPR ($r = -0.79$; $p = 0.004$), and visual recognition response time and TPR ($r = 0.61$; $p = 0.046$). The results of this study indicate that the highest ranked tennis players possessed the best VEPT scores, highest VEPT rank, most correct visual tracking percent, and fastest visual recognition response time. The results of this study indicate a significant positive relationship between visual skills and tennis performance of NCAA Division I tennis players. Subsequently, coaches may consider using visual skills programs such as VEPT to assess and train tennis athletes.

Spaniol et al., (2011) to investigate the relationship between visual skills and volleyball performance of NCAA Division I volleyball players. Participants consisted of thirteen female NCAA Division I volleyball players (height 179.36 ± 7.73cm, age 18-25 years) who were evaluated for visual skills and performance during the 2008-2009 seasons. Subjects were assessed for eye alignment, depth perception, convergence, divergence, visual recognition, and visual tracking. A composite score (final VEPT score) was also calculated for each subject. Volleyball performance was determined by end of season statistics, which included kills, kills per set, attack errors, hitting percentage, assists, assists per set, serve aces, serve aces per set, serve errors, reception errors, digs, digs per set, blocks solo, blocks assisted, total blocks, blocks per set, blocking errors, and ball-handling errors. Data analysis was performed by utilizing a correlation matrix to calculate correlation coefficients between the vision and performance variables. Statistical analysis indicated significant ($p < 0.05$) relationships between convergence percentage and attack percentage ($r = 0.55$), divergence station score and assists per set (r = 0.53), visual recognition percent correct and hitting percentage (r = 0.71), eye alignment and blocks per set (r = -0.56), visual recognition response time and attack percentage (r = -0.74), and visual recognition percent correct and reception errors (r = - 0.57). The results of this study indicate that superior visual skills were highly related to superior volleyball performance statistics in several areas. Since visual skills appear to play a crucial role in volleyball performance, coaches may consider using programs such as VEPT to assess volleyball players.

Fowler and Toit (2009) to achieve their greatest potentials, aspects of sport such as reaction time and hand-eye co-ordination needs to be at their peaks. Sports vision aims to enhance performance through a variety of procedures and training techniques. Rugby players aged 18 to 26 were subjected to a sports vision battery consisting of three different hand-eye co-ordination tests. An improvement in performance was observed by players exposed to the exercises. In the „number of catches" test there was a meaningful improvement of 12%. A 22% improvement was observed in the number of successful catches (simultaneous ball- throwing) and an 8% and 3% improvement in the number of successful throws through a ring (accurate passing) to the left and right sides respectively. It is very important to measure hand-eye co-ordination alongside the standard measuring of cardiopulmonary and metabolic status to determine the athletic abilities of sporting individuals. Visual abilities can affect both motor skill and performance. This study proves that correct training programs and hand-eye co-ordination tests can vastly improve sporting performance. Athletes are advised to complete at least 15 minutes of sport-specific visual training during each day of practice.

Toit et al., (2009) to determine the visual skills of soccer players by assessing depth perception, accommodation flexibility, eye tracking, eye jumps, peripheral awareness and visual memory of soccer players. Forty-eight soccer players aged 12 to 20 were assessed. The results were compared according to age group and the four main positions in soccer, namely: striker, midfielder, defender and goalkeeper. The results indicated that visual skills tend to improve with age and that different positions do not necessarily require different levels of visual skills. This reinforces the suggestion that visual skills are not necessarily a function of the position one plays. Sportsmen will have a great advantage over their fellow rivals due to improvements in their exercise and sports vision training programs. These training programs can help improve and train the athlete"s visual coordination, increase concentration and focus, hand-eye co-ordination, anticipation as well as gain knowledge about their motor response. These principles can also be implemented in a similar evaluation of other athletes and non-athletes.

Planer (1994) explained that the quick identification of objects as they move through space rely on aspects of eye movements, focus flexibility, fusion flexibility and depth perception. The author explained that these relates to the ability of the eyes to work together when watching a moving object, to quickly and simultaneously change focus with minimum effort, to fuse these objects together, and then to use these clear fused images quickly so as to perceive depth.

Ward and Williams (2000) many visual variables have been investigated with respect to their contribution to motor skill and sporting performance. The authors explain that given the nature of soccer performance, variables such as acuity, depth perception, and peripheral awareness are all potential factors which may contribute to the accurate detection and reception of information upon which game winning decisions can be made. It is postulated that in soccer, a combination of these functions, in varying degrees, is necessary for players to meet visual demands and efficiently fulfill their role.

Pearson (2004) pointed out that once programmed agility drills "are learnt and performed on a regular basis, times and performances will improve and advances in strength, explosion, flexibility and body control will be witnessed". The author stated that random agility drills are the most difficult to master, prepare for and perform. Here the coach can incorporate visual and audible reactive skills so that the cricket and soccer player has to make split-second decisions with movements based upon the various stimuli.

Twist and Benicky (1996) has found that for continued progression, the coach must incorporate visual stimulus. For cricket and soccer players, this involves catching tennis balls during off-field drills or receiving a pass during complex movements on the field. These types of drills remain constant in that the player always knows where to go and when to expect the ball. These authors found that next the coach can incorporate some visual or auditory stimulus in varied movement patterns. Players may explode into action after a ball is dropped in front of them, to either catch it before it hits the ground again or kick the ball on the bounce (soccer). Coaches can also call out directions (auditory stimulus). These types of drills are "react and explode" drills, where the cricket and soccer players have to react and, with body control, co-ordinate the movement, and quickly explode to a certain direction

McCarthy (1996) designing any type of strength, conditioning, speed, and agility programme, a coach must first assess the unique demands of the sports in question – not only the physiological demands but also what is required in strength, agility, flexibility, and balance. By training fast, the players become faster in their movements. if all of their movements in a game are fast reactive movements, it makes sense to train in this way. It is due to this statement that sprinters train to be fast obviously and they only train in a manner that enhances their fast twitch muscle fibres. By training the player"s anaerobic-fitness energy system, the player will be way ahead of his opposition, as they will still be training in a way that is not allowing them to display their full cricketing potential.

Knudson and Kluka (1997) although physical education teachers and coaches are aware of safety procedures and protective equipment for the eyes in many sports, many may not be aware of facts about human vision that are relevant to sport. Visual abilities affect sport performance and the acquisition of motor skills, and can be improved with training. This article summarizes important vision information related to performance in sport, shows how teachers can easily use vision training to improve performance, and provides practical examples of applying this knowledge in teaching.

Elmurr et al. (1996) has found that the game of table tennis, and many other sports that are involved in detecting any fast moving object, requires the execution of extremely precise sensor motor skills to allow the athlete to compete at an elite level. It is postulated that saccadic eye movements play an important role in the execution of these sensor motor tasks. According to these authors the duration of the reaction time of saccadic eye movement are longer than the actual saccade duration. Changes in the saccadic reaction time may be more significant than the change in duration. Therefore, it would appear that the saccadic reaction time is the most crucial saccadic parameter that may influence an athlete"s total reaction time.

Wood et al., (1994) Vision training programmes offered by general optometrists are claimed to be extremely effective and are being increasingly used by a large range of sports teams and even individual athletes. In the past it is found that the question that was examined experimentally was whether such programmes really work, in improving both the athlete"s vision and performance, or whether the claims for their efficiency in improving sports performance are unfounded.

Manuel et al., (2007) to evaluate visual abilities such as distance visual acuity, binocular horizontal visual field, simple and choice visual reaction times, and stereoscopic vision in skilled 11- to 13-yr.-old basketball players participating in a 15-day summer training camp. On a test battery, visual abilities were monitored in 473 players of the Spanish Basketball Federation over a 5-yr. period. The players showed outstanding scores on distance visual acuity and stereoscopic vision, and good visual reaction times and horizontal visual fields. When scores were compared by sex and age, significant differences on certain visual measures were observed. Many players showed crossed eye-hand dominance. Visual screening programs may help promote visual health among junior basketball players and could be used for performance training.

Bennett and Davids (1995) studied the available information for controlling a multi degree-of-freedom sport action was manipulated in 2 experiments. In the first, 10 intermediate lifters were participants; for the second, 8 skilled and 8 less skilled lifters were observed. Three single repetitions of a power lift squat were performed under 3 vision conditions (i.e., full, ambient, no vision). The less skilled and intermediate lifters' technical performance decreased significantly with the removal of visual information. There was no detrimental effect in the skilled group. Despite the differing information constraints, skilled lifters exhibited a high level of positioning accuracy and timing consistency across conditions. These data fail to support the theoretical predictions of the specificity of learning hypothesis. The differences between the task constraints in this study and those in manual aiming investigations may represent a boundary to the current propositions of the specificity of learning hypothesis.

Montes et al., (2000) to investigate the eye-hand and eye-foot visual reaction time among young soccer players and to compare those with non-soccer players in order to evaluate possible differences. A vision screening of 53 young male soccer players belonging to the Valencia Soccer Club was done. Soccer players were divided in three categories, with mean ages of 8.2 0.5 years (range, 8- to 9-year olds), 10.6 0.2 years (range, 10- to 11-year-olds), and 12.7 0.3 years (range, 12- to 13-year-olds). An age-matched sample of 60 young male non-soccer players served as a control population. Mean ages in this population were 8.3 0.6 years, 10.5 0.4 years, and 12.6 0.2 years for each category, respectively. Eye-hand and eye-foot visual reaction times were determined in players and non-players by means of a computer-controlled stimuli device. There are statistically significant differences between eye-hand and eye-foot reaction times between players and non players (p 0.05). Eye-hand and eye-foot visual reaction times were found to be different between the two populations evaluated. The results show differences between soccer and non-soccer players, with the soccer players demonstrating faster reaction times.

Dane and Ali (2003) conducted a study on sex and handedness differences in the eye-dominant hand, the right eye-right hand and the left eye-left hand visual reaction times were studied in 270 right-handed and 56 left-handed young handball players. Reaction time was assessed by a software package. All visual reaction times were longer in women than in men. In the eye-dominant hand and the left eye- left hand visual reaction times, the left-handers had superiority over the right handers, but there was no difference between the right eye-right hand visual reaction times of the right- and left-handers. In right-handers, all visual reaction times were longer in women than in men, but there was no sex difference in left-handers. The results suggest that left-handed players have probably an intrinsic neurological advantage.

Dane et al., (2008) examined the relations of simple reaction times of right and left hands with muscle powers of right and left hands, back, and leg were. Hand preference was assessed by the modified Edinburgh Handedness Inventory. The simple reaction time (SRT) for right hand was not correlated with right and left hand and leg. The left hand SRT was significantly negatively correlated with right and left hand and leg powers. The choice RT was significantly correlated with right and left hand powers, but not leg power. There were no right-left differences in simple RT and hand power. These results suggest that sport activities are associated with eye-hand visual reaction time (VRT) and visuospatial intelligence (VSI). Exercise's positive effect may be associated with especially the right brain or left hand.

Spaniol et al., (2011) to investigate the relationship between visual skills and volleyball performance of NCAA Division I volleyball players. Participants consisted of thirteen female NCAA Division I volleyball players (height 179.36 ± 7.73cm, age 18-25 years) who were evaluated for visual skills and performance during the 2008-2009 season. Visual skills were assessed using Visual Edge Performance Trainer® (VEPT), a commercial software program designed to evaluate and train visual skills. Subjects were assessed for eye alignment, depth perception, convergence, divergence, visual recognition, and visual tracking. A composite score (final VEPT score) was also calculated for each subject. Volleyball performance was determined by end of season statistics, which included kills, kills per set, attack errors, hitting percentage, assists, assists per set, serve aces, serve aces per set, serve errors, reception errors, digs, digs per set, blocks solo, blocks assisted, total blocks, blocks per set, blocking errors, and ball-handling errors. Data analysis was performed by utilizing a correlation matrix to calculate correlation coefficients between the vision and performance variables. The results of this study indicate that superior visual skills were highly related to superior volleyball performance statistics in several areas. Since visual skills appear to play a crucial role in volleyball performance, coaches may consider using programs such as VEPT to assess volleyball players.

Marina et al., (2010) to define which coordination abilities are the most important in tennis and to evaluate whether a coordination training program will improve the service technique. The study was conducted on 48 children (age 11 ± 2 years). The participants were randomly divided into a control group (C) and an intervention group (A) that performed a specific coordination program 3 times/wk. Both groups (C and A) followed a tennis training program 3times/wk. The service technique was evaluated in all subjects in the beginning of the protocol (T0), after the completion of the 5-week specific coordination program (T5) and one week after the intervention program was completed (T6). The present study, suggests that the most important coordination abilities for tennis players are kinaesthetic differentiation and reaction time. Furthermore, two-way repeated measurements ANOVA revealed that there was significant increase (p _0.05) on the service technique between groups (C and A) and among the different phases (T0, T5 and T6).

Wimshurst et al., (2012) Many sports require fine spatiotemporal resolution for optimal performance. Previous studies have compared anticipatory skills and the decision-making process in athletes; however, there is little information on visual skills of elite athletes, particularly hockey players. To assess visual skills of Olympic hockey players and analyze differences by playing position, and to analyze improvement of visual skills after training, 21 Olympic field hockey players were pre- and post-tested on 11 visual tasks following a 10-wk. visual training program consisting of computer-based visual exercises. There were no mean differences at pre-test between players of different positions, suggesting that performance on these visual skills was independent of playing position. However, after training, an improvement was seen in all players (when scores were averaged across all 11 visual tasks) with goalkeepers improving significantly more than any other position. This suggests the possibility of improving visual skills even in an elite population.

Abdullah et al., (2009) to compare the visual skills of expert and novice soccer referees. Twenty expert soccer referees, twenty two novice soccer referees and twenty non-athletes male students were investigated for facility of accommodation, peripheral vision, eye saccadic movements and speed of recognition. The results showed that the expert soccer referees were superior in all of the visual skills, but there was no significant difference between novice referees and non-athletes. This substantial difference between expert and novice soccer referees implies that these visual skills are important for refereeing soccer. For detecting other visual skills in soccer, referees must use visual skills from other programs. This study suggested that talent identification and development of visual abilities among soccer referees is of fundamental importance to success.

Ashraf and Ahmed (2010) to design a training program of complex skills and vision drills for improving velocity and accuracy of motor performance for complex skills with ball, also to identify the effect of vision training program on developing skilled performance and the improving ratios in foot player juniors. A total of 30 football players, 16years old, 15 years old, as added subjects, not included in the main research population, to ensure quality of Procedure from 8-6-2008 to 11-6-2008, to determine the heart pulses pre performance as an indicator for recovery, after 90-120 seconds rest, with 75-85 pulse average per minute. As well as to find out the correct distance for the player to execute different motor combinations. The suggested training program and vision drills showed a positive effect on velocity and accuracy of motor performance of complex skills with ball, developing visual ability in football juniors. Results showed statistical significant differences between pre-post measures, on quick motor performance of complex skills with ball, as well as improving ratios, for the post measure.

Schorer and Baker (2009) to determine whether the perceptual-motor abilities of highly skilled performers in dynamic, time-constrained sports exhibited the same pattern of age-related decline seen in other areas. The sample for this study involved five age-specific groups of handball goalkeepers. Each participant completed an eye-tracking task, a temporal occlusion task, and an eight-choice reaction time task. Results revealed age-related declines in motor performance but not perceptual performance. Skilled perception appears resistant to normal age-related declines over time through the use of compensatory mechanisms.

Ghasemi et al., (2011) previous studies have compared visual skills of expert and novice athletes; referees' performance has not been addressed. Visual skills of two groups of expert referees, successful and unsuccessful in decision making, were compared. Using video clips of soccer matches to assess decision-making success of 41 national and international referees from 31 to 42 years of age, 10 top referees were selected as the Successful group and 10 as the Unsuccessful group. Visual tests included visual memory, visual reaction time, peripheral vision, recognition speed, saccadic eye movement, and facility of accommodation. The Successful group had better visual skills than the Unsuccessful group. Such visual skills enhance soccer referees' performance and may be recommended for young referees.

Jafarzadehpur et, al., (2007) interaction of sport exercise and visual functions. Some aspects of visual skills have been evaluated in volleyball players. Eighty-three normal females were categorized in four groups; non-players (NP), beginner volleyball players, intermediate and advanced players. Facility of accommodation and far saccade for autotypes at three distances were measured. The athletes showed better facility of accommodation and saccadic eye movement (SEM) than the non-playing control group. There was a significant difference (P<0.001) between NP and beginner players with advanced players and intermediate players. There are mutual interrelations between the visual system and sensory-motor coordination of the whole body. In a "programmed" activity many motor and sensorial elements interactively influence one another. The visual system, as the most important coordinator, navigates the "programmed" activities. The facility of accommodation shows how fast clear vision can be accomplished. The saccadic eye movement shows how fast visual system can fixate on an object. Improvement of these two parameters indicates that the visual system can change fixation very fast and clearly see a new fixation point promptly. These are the requirement for a good volleyball player; hence, we find better visual performance in advanced players than in others.

Sarpeshkar and Mann (2011) Cricket batting is an incredibly complex task which requires the coordination of full-body movements to successfully hit a fast moving ball. Biomechanical studies on batting have helped to shed light on how this intricate skill may be performed, yet the many different techniques exhibited by batters make the systematic examination of batting difficult. This review seeks to critically evaluate the existing literature examining cricket batting, but doing so by exploring the strong but often neglected relationship between biomechanics and visual motor control. In three separate sections, the paper seeks to address (i) the different theories of motor control which may help to explain how skilled batters can hit a ball, (ii) strategies used by batters to overcome the (at times excessive) temporal constraints, and (iii) an interpretation from a visual-motor perspective of the prevailing biomechanical data on batting.

Roberts et al., (2010) examined the interactive effects of different visual imagery perspectives and narcissism on motor performance. In both studies participants completed the Narcissistic Personality Inventory (NPI-40: Raskin & Hall, 1979) and were assigned to either an internal visual imagery or external visual imagery group. Participants then performed a motor task (dart throwing in Study 1 and golf putting in Study 2) under conditions of practice, low self-enhancement, and high self-enhancement. Following completion of the respective tasks, participants were categorized into high and low narcissistic groups based on their NPI-40 scores. In both studies, high narcissists using external visual imagery significantly improved performance from the low to the high self-enhancement condition, whereas high narcissists using internal visual imagery did not. Low narcissists remained relatively constant in performance across self-enhancement conditions, regardless of perspective. The results highlight the importance of considering personality characteristics when examining the effects of visual imagery perspectives on performance.

Stine et al., (1982) studied on visual abilities to enhance sports performance is explored. Optometric intervention in sports assumes the following statements to be true: Athletes have better visual abilities than non-athletes and better athletes have better visual abilities than the poorer athletes, Visual abilities are trainable, and Visual training is transferable to the performance of the athlete. The literature demonstrates that athletes have better visual abilities than non-athletes. Studies have shown this to be true in the following areas of vision: Larger extent of visual fields, larger fields of recognition (peripheral acuity), larger motion perception fields, lower amounts of heterophoria at near and far, more consistent simultaneous vision, more accurate depth perception, better dynamic visual acuity, and better ocular motilities. The literature also shows that all of the above skills are trainable. Two studies are cited that support the belief that visual training is transferable to athletic performance but they suffer from inadequate experimental design.

Müller and Abernethy (2006) Studied the capability of cricket batsmen of different skill levels to pick-up information from the pre-release movement pattern of the bowler, from pre-bounce ball flight, and from post-bounce ball flight was examined experimentally. Six highly skilled and six low-skilled cricket batsmen batted against three different leg-spin bowlers while wearing liquid crystal spectacles. The spectacles permitted the specific information available to the batsmen on each trial to be manipulated such that vision was either: (i) occluded at a point prior to the point of ball release (thereby only allowing vision of advance information from the bowler's delivery action); (ii) occluded at a point prior to the point of ball bounce (thereby permitting the additional vision of pre-bounce ball flight); or (iii) not occluded (thereby permitting the additional vision of post-bounce ball flight information). Measurement was made on each trial of both the accuracy of the definitive (forward-backward) foot movements made by the batsmen and their success (or otherwise) in making bat-ball contact. The analyses revealed a superior capability of the more skilled players to make use of earlier (pre-bounce) ball flight information to guide successful bat-ball interception, thus mirroring the greater use of prospective information pick-up by skilled performers observed in other aspects of batting and in other time-constrained performance domains.

McLeod (1978) suggest that some aspects of high-speed ball games such as cricket are 'impossible' because there is insufficient time for the player to respond to unpredictable movements of the ball. Given the success with which some people perform these supposedly impossible acts, it has been assumed by some commentators that laboratory measures of reaction time are not applicable to skilled performers. An analysis of high-speed film of international cricketers batting on a specially prepared pitch which produced unpredictable movement of the ball is reported, and it is shown that, when batting, highly skilled professional cricketers show reaction times of around 200 ms, times similar to those found in traditional laboratory studies. Furthermore, professional cricketers take roughly as long as casual players to pick up ball flight information from film of bowlers. These two sets of results suggest that the dramatic contrast between the ability of skilled and unskilled sportsmen to act on the basis of visual information does not lie in differences in the speed of operation of the perceptual system. It lies in the organization of the motor system that uses the output of the perceptual system.

CHAPTER III
METHODOLOGY

CHAPTER - III

METHODOLOGY

In this chapter, the selection of subjects, selection of variables, selection of the tests, reliability of the instruments, reliability of data, testers" competency, orientation of subjects, test administration, training programme, experimental design, collection of data and statistical procedures have been explained.

3.1 Selection of Subjects

The purpose of the present study was to find out the effect of visual skill fitness training on selected visual skills and skill related fitness variables of male cricket players. To achieve this purpose, as subjects, one hundred and thirty four (N = 134) cricket players were selected as subjects. The selected subjects were the players pertained to teams qualified for quarterfinals in inter-collegiate level tournament. The subjects selected for this study were hailed from various socio-economic conditions. Their age was fixed in the range of 19 – 24 years.

3.2 Selection of Variables

Visual involvement in a sport varies according to environmental demands associated with that sport. These environmental demands are matched by a task specific motor response. In order to measure the athletic ability of a cricket player it is important not only to measure the physical skills of the player, but also the visual skills. The importance of coaching or training the players in cricket has been heavily reliant upon repetition of motor skills, conditioning and weight training. Although strength and endurance are beneficial to the sport and can still be conducted without guidance by a coaching authority, repetition of motor skills is the key to any individual or team success and it should always be monitored to ensure that the skill is being repeated correctly. In such a way the need of visual skill fitness training in sport is a value added one as it stretches the performance of a player positively. Hence to complicate the VSFT in cricket, and to study its effect, the variables related visual skill and performance were identifies. Thus, the selected variables are: eye-hand co-ordination, visual reaction time and depth perception was chosen as (visual skills), arm explosive power, leg explosive power, speed, agility and balance was chosen as (skill related fitness variables).

3.3 Tools used in the Study

The researcher had consulted with experts, Physical Education Professionals and reviewed various literatures and selected the following standardized tests, which are appropriate and ideal to measure the selected variables. The criterion variables are presented in Table – 3.1.

Table 3.1

Tests Selection

S. No	Variables	Tests	Unit of measurements
	Visual skill Variables		
1	Hand-eye co-ordination	Mirror tracing test	In Numbers
2	Visual reaction time	Chronoscope	In seconds
3	Depth perception	Depth perception apparatus	In centimeters
	Skill related fitness variables		
4	Arm explosive power	Seated medicine ball throw	In meters
5	Leg explosive power	Sergeant vertical Jump	In centimeters
6	Speed	50 Yards Dash	In seconds
7	Agility	Illinois agility test	In seconds
8	Balance	Stork balance stand test	In seconds

3.4 Experimental Design

In this study pre post random of experiment design was used. From the selected samples (N = 134) using conventional sampling method, thirty subjects were randomly selected. They were assigned equally into two groups namely Visual Skill Fitness Training Group (VSFTG) and control group (CG). The Visual Skill Fitness Training Group (VSFTG) underwent scientifically designed training program of VSFT training program for two days a week for about twelve weeks. Subjects of control group is concerned, they were also engaged into their own training schedule in the game of cricket. They were instructed to keep off them from any specific training that develops the visual skills. Thus finally 30 subjects were taken for the present study. All the subjects gave written informed consent and no compulsion was made to take part in the training programme and the subjects were free to withdraw their consent in case of feeling any discomfort during the period of their participation but there was no drop out during the study. A qualified physician examined the subjects and declared that they were medically and physically fit to participate in the training programme.

3.5 Reliabity of Data

The reliability of data was measured by ensuring instruments" reliability, tester"s competency and subject"s reliability.

3.5.1 Instruments" Reliability

With respect to the instruments used in measuring variables, certificate of accuracy was obtained from appropriate instruments" testing agency, and also by recalibrating the scale using known amounts of variables wherever required.

Table - 3.2

Reliability Coefficients of Test Retest Scores of Criterion Variables

S. No.	Criterion Variables	" r " Value
1	Mirror tracing	0.88
2	Chronoscope	0.98
3	Depth perception	0.85
4	Seated medicine ball throw	0.92
5	Vertical jump	0.94
6	50yards dash	0.94
7	Illinois agility test	0.93
8	Stroke balance	0.97

3.5.2 Tester's Competency

The assistance of two specially trained physical education teachers was sought on administration of various test items. They were oriented about the procedures of measuring and recording the scores in each variable. All the assistants were asked to measure on a few subjects and co-efficient of inter correlation of scores recorded by them were taken. The final measuring programme was conducted only on getting high co-efficient of correlation.

3.5.3 Orientation of the Subjects

The investigator explained the purpose of the study to the subjects clearly. Instructions in connection with the testing procedure while measuring the selected variables were also explained to the subjects. Three sessions were spent to familiarize the subjects with the technique involved in various tests used to collect the data.

3.6 Pilot Study

The present study was mainly concerned with the effects of Visual skill fitness training on selected visual skills and skill related fitness variables of male cricket players. The type of training used in the present study was Visual Skill Fitness Training. Earlier But the present study was mainly concerned with visual skill fitness training. For this purpose, the investigator conducted a pilot study, for which 20 inter- collegiate cricket players were selected as sample for the pilot study. They were assigned to treatment specifically designed for the presents study such as visual skill fitness training on selected visual skills and skill related fitness variables of male cricket players.

3.7 TEST ADMINISTRATION

3.7.1 Eye-Hand Co-ordination

It is the ability to measure the eye-hand co-ordination of an individual by using mirror tracing test. The tracing mirror was placed safely on the table. A bell was attached to the tracing mirror. Concentration was given to the plus point. To find out the eye-hand co-ordination, the subjects were asked to move the tracing needle through the tracing mirror. If the needle touches on the wire while moving, the bell rings. Foul should be counted according to the alarm sound. Ten trials were given to all subjects. An average score of all trials was taken as score for calculation.

3.7.2 Visual Reaction Time Test

It is the ability to measure the visual reaction time of an individual by using Chronoscope. The instrument consists of a wooden board with a screen in the middle. On one side of the screen (The subjects side), there is one red light and two press keys. The keys are connected to the light. If the key is pressed while the light is burning, the circuit will automatically break and the light will go off. On the other side, (i.e.) the tester"s side, there is a series of keys which serve to switch on the red light on the subject"s side.

3.7.3 Depth Perception

The subject was asked to sit in front of the depth perception apparatus. The subject was asked to ensure that the three rods existing in the box would be in a line. Then the investigator changed the position of two rods that were on either side of apparatus. On the signal to start, the investigator moved the two rods that were in lateral side towards the rod in the centre. Then the subject was instructed to use the command „stop" when he identified the three rods that were in line. On the command of the subject, the distance to the centre is considered as score of the depth perception.

3.7.4 Arm Explosive power (Seated Medicine ball Throw)

The arm explosive power of the player was measured by using the chair sitting two-kilo gram medicine ball throw. The thrown distance was measured in meters and recorded as the score.

3.7.5 Leg Explosive Power (Vertical Jump)

The leg explosive power was measured by the vertical jump with the help of the stand and reach test (Chu, 1996). The vertical jump test was completed from a 2-foot standing position without a step into the jump. The subject was asked to stand with side to the wall keeping both feet flat on the floor. He reached as high as possible with his middle finger touching the wall. This was his standing reach. Keeping color chalk powder on his middle finger he stood comfortable at a distance from the wall. On signal the subject swung both arms upward and jumped vertically extending his hand and touching the wall with the chalked finger. This jump must be taken without any preliminary feet movement such as hopping or stepping. The difference between standing hand reach and the jump reach were recorded. Out of three attempts the best reach was taken and recorded.

3.7.6 50 Yards Dash

The 50 yards dash was used to measure speed **(AAHPER Youth Fitness Test Manual 1975)**. In this test, the subjects (two at a time) stood behind the starting time. On getting a signal (the clap), the subjects ran as fast as possible across the finishing line. Finally the scoring of this test item is the time elapsed between the start and the moment the subject crosses the finish line. It was recorded to the nearest one-tenth of a second.

3.7.7 Illinois Agility Test

Illinois agility test is a commonly used test for measure agility. The aim of the test is to complete a weaving running course in the shortest possible time. Equipments required was flat non-slip surface, marking cones and stopwatch and, Measuring tape. The length of the course is 10 meters and the width (distance between the start and finish points) is 5 meters. Four cones are used to mark the start, finish and the two turning points. Another four cones are placed down the center an equal distance apart. Each cone in the center is spaced 3.3 meters apart.

The subject starts face down, with the head to the start line, and hands by the shoulders. At the whistle, the subject ran the course, without knocking down any cones. Scoring is the time elapsed between the starting and finishing point was recorded to the one-tenth of a second **(Getchell, 1979).**

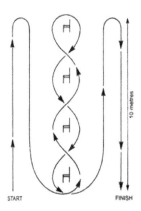

3.7.8 Stork Balance Stand Test

To assess the ability to balance on the ball of the foot. Remove the shoes and place the hands on the hips, then position the non-supporting foot against the inside knee of the supporting leg. The subject is given one minute to practice the balance. The subject raises the heel to balance on the ball of the foot. The stopwatch is started as the heel is raised from the floor. The stopwatch is stopped if any of the follow occurs: the hand(s) come off the hips. The supporting foot swivels or moves (hops) in any direction. The non-supporting foot loses contact with the knee. The heel of the supporting foot touches the floor. The total time in seconds is recorded. The score is the best of three attempts (Johnson and Nelson, 1979).

3.8 COLLECTION OF DATA – Pre-test

To study the base line performance of subjects belongs to Visual Skill Fitness Training (VSFTG), and Control Group (CG) on variables such as eye-hand co-ordination, visual reaction time and depth perception (visual skills variables), arm explosive power, leg explosive power, speed, agility and balance (skill related fitness variables) used in the study, the subjects of each group were measured using the standardized tests as mentioned earlier. The performances of subjects of both groups on variables are considered as pre-test score.

3.9 ADMINISTRATION OF TRAINING PROGRAMME

The procedure adopted in the training programme for the present study is described below:-

1. During the training period, Group-I underwent Visual Skill Fitness Training Programme and Group - II served as a control group they did not involved in any specific training programme. Other than the training program they undergone traditionally.

2. The intensity for the Visual Skill Fitness Training Programme (VSFTP - Group I), was fixed on the basis of the results of the pilot study, and

3. The Visual Skill Fitness Training Programme was carried out at Karunya University, Coimbatore, Tamil Nadu. The subjects of experimental group underwent their respective training programmers for two days a week for twelve weeks under the supervision researcher in morning sessions. In the evening session all the subjects were engaged with their regular practices.

3.10 TRAINING PROCEDURE

The procedure used for the visual skill fitness training (VSFT) is as follows. The total duration of VSFT was 12 weeks. These twelve weeks VSFT was segmented into three phases. The duration of training programme for each phase was four week. Thus the Phase – 1 was executed in first four weeks (1st, 2nd, 3rd & 4th), Phase – 2 was executed in the second four weeks (5th, 6th, 7th & 8th) and the Phase – 3 was executed in the third four weeks (9th, 10th, 11th & 12th).

Visual skill fitness training programme administered for subjects for two days a week for about 12 weeks. The duration of training for a day was 60 - 75 minutes. Of this 10 minutes used for warm – up, 5 minutes used for cool down.

The detailed and structure of for VSFT programs 45 – 60 minutes for three phases are described as follows.

3.10.1 Phase - I   First four week Training Program

In this phase subjects of VSFT were treated with running drills and visual skills station for 45 - 60 minutes. Subjects of this VSFT group were started with first running station after completion of running drills which they moved into visual skill training stations. In these training program nine exercises was fixed. Thus, seven running stations and two visual skill station were used during this programme. 3 sets were fixed for the first four week training programme. Duration of exercise in station was fixed for 30 seconds, the rest in between the station was fixed for 30 seconds and rest in between sets was fixed for 3 minutes.

Table - 3.3

Phase - I   First four week Training Program

Stations	S. No	Exercises	Duration of exercise in station	No of Sets	Rest in between station	Rest in between sets
Running drills	1	Speed - and - Agility	30 seconds	3	30 seconds	3 minutes
	2	x4 Push-ups – x4 Shuttles	30 seconds	3	30 seconds	3 minutes
	3	Carioca	30 seconds	3	30 seconds	3 minutes
	4	S - Touch – R	30 seconds	3	30 seconds	3 minutes
	5	Medicine Ball - Forward Throw	30 seconds	3	30 seconds	3 minutes
	6	S ½ - R - S - P – R	30 seconds	3	30 seconds	3 minutes
	7	Shuffel Drill	30 seconds	3	30 seconds	3 minutes
Visual skills	1	Push-Up and Catch	30 seconds	3	30 seconds	3 minutes
	2	Simultaneous Ball Throw	30 seconds	3	30 seconds	3 minutes

S – Sprint Forward, **R** – Running Backwards, **P** - Push – up

3.10.2 Phase - II   Second four week Training Program

In this phase subjects of VSFT were treated with running and visual skill station for 45- 60 minutes. Subjects of this VSFT group were started with first running station after completion of running drills which they moved into visual skill training stations. In these training program nine exercises was fixed. Thus, five running stations and four visual skill station were used during this programme. 4 sets were fixed for the first four week training programme. Duration of exercise in station was fixed for 30 seconds, the rest in between the station was fixed for 30 seconds and rest in between sets was fixed for 3 minutes.

Table - 3.4

Phase - II   Second four week Training Program

Stations	S. No	Exercises	Duration of exercise in station	No of Sets	Rest in between station	Rest in between sets
Running drills	1	S – P – R	30 seconds	4	30 seconds	3 minutes
	2	S ½ x4 - S - P – R	30 seconds	4	30 seconds	3 minutes
	3	Static Hold and Run	30 seconds	4	30 seconds	3 minutes
	4	Ladder Work	30 seconds	4	30 seconds	3 minutes
	5	S ½ - P - S - P – R	30 seconds	4	30 seconds	3 minutes
Visual skills	1	2 Vs 1	30 seconds	4	30 seconds	3 minutes
	2	Box Drill – Call	30 seconds	4	30 seconds	3 minutes
	3	Box Drill – Throw	30 seconds	4	30 seconds	3 minutes
	4	Crucifix Ball Drop	30 seconds	4	30 seconds	3 minutes

S – Sprint Forward

R – Running Backwards

P - Push – up

3.10.3 Phase - III   Third four week Training Program

In this phase subjects of VSFT were treated with running and visual skill station for 45 – 60 minutes. Subjects of this VSFT group were started with first running station after completion of running drills which they moved into visual skill training stations. In these training program ten exercises was fixed. Thus, three running stations and six visual skill station were used during this programme. 5 sets were fixed for the first four week training programme. Duration of exercise in station was fixed for 30 seconds, the rest in between the station was fixed for 30 seconds and rest in between sets was fixed for 3 minutes.

Table - 3.5

Phase - III   Third four week Training Program

Stations	S. No	Exercises	Duration of exercise in station	No of Sets	Rest in between station	Rest in between sets
Running drills	1	S ½ - P - S - turn - S ½ - P - S	30 seconds	5	30 seconds	3 minutes
	2	Medicine Ball - Backwards Throw	30 seconds	5	30 seconds	3 minutes
	3	Static Hold on a Gym Ball	30 seconds	5	30 seconds	3 minutes
Visual skills	1	Lateral Shuffle and Ball Catch	30 seconds	5	30 seconds	3 minutes
	2	2 Vs 1 – Variation	30 seconds	5	30 seconds	3 minutes
	3	Chasers	30 seconds	5	30 seconds	3 minutes
	4	Lateral Shuffle and ball Change	30 seconds	5	30 seconds	3 minutes
	5	Ladder Work with Balls	30 seconds	5	30 seconds	3 minutes
	6	T-Drill	30 seconds	5	30 seconds	3 minutes

S – Sprint Forward
R – Running Backwards
P - Push – up

3.11   Description for running drills

Speed – and – Agility

The researcher placed 2 beacons approximately 20 m apart, the subjects must run the 20 m ten times. The subject must try and do this 50 seconds and this drill must be performed twice.

Sprint forward – Push-ups – Backward Running

The researcher placed Place 2 beacons approximately 20 m apart. The Subject should sprint forward complete one push-up at the 20 m mark. Explode up from push-up and run backwards to starting point, and continue this drill until the time is over.

Static Hold and Run

The Subject should start in a static-hold (bridge) position. On the researcher demand "go" the subjects jump up and run shuttles. Keep on running until researcher says "hold", where the subjects go back to starting line and hold position until "go" Hold the position for 5-7 sec and then say "go".

Shuffel Drill

When the researcher says "ready" they immediately have to start moving their feet on the spot (running on the spot). A "ready" position is when the subject"s hands are up knees bent and subject mimic a basketball subject"s body language. When they hear "side" they have to jump sideways in the direction that the researcher is pointing and continue to move their feet, head up and hands forward and palms pointing forward. When the researcher says "twist" they perform a twisting action with their hips (in the direction that the researcher is pointing) when they have mastered this combine the "side" and the "twist".

Sprint forward – Push-ups – Backward running ½ - S – P – S

The Subjects should sprint forward (20 m) go down and complete one push-up. Explode up from push-up and run backwards to the middle beacon. The touch the "line" and sprint forward again do another push-up. Explode up from push-up and sprint back to starting point.

x4 Push-ups – x4 Shuttles

The Subjects should start with x4 push-ups, jump up, sprint to the 20 m mark, Touch the "line" and sprint back, complete x4 shuttle runs.

Ladder Work

The Subject should starts on the side of the ladder. The aim is to develop linear fast feet with control, precision and power. It is very important that the subjects move with fast and quick feet through the ladder. Run with one foot in each block and run with both feet in each block. When the subject gets to the end of the ladder. He runs back to the start and continues with the sequence.

Carioca

The Subjects should cover the length of the grid by moving laterally. The rear foot crosses in front of the body and then moves around to the back simultaneously the lead foot does the opposite. The arms also move across the front and back of the body. The aim is to improve hip mobility and speed. This will increase the firing of nerve impulse over a period of time to develop balance and co-ordination while moving and twisting.

Medicine Ball – Forward Throw

The Subject should stand on his knees in an up-right position. Hold medicine ball above and slightly behind his head and bend arms backwards by dropping the ball slightly and move slightly backwards from the knees upwards to gain momentum. Extend arms forward and throw the ball. Almost like a two-hand over head throw the Subject must try to throw ball as far as possible.

Medicine Ball – Backwards Throw

The Subject should stands with his back to his partner. The ball is on the ground in front of him Subject place his hands on the sides of the ball and with bent knees, Lift the ball up, bend arms and throw the ball backwards over his head. Extend arms when the ball is released. Important that the subject extend his legs when releasing the ball. The Subject must try to throw ball as far as possible.

Sprint forward – touch – Backward Running

The Subject should sprint forward up to the 20 m mark. Touch the "line" with two hands. Important that the subject bends his knees when touching the line and head must be up. Run backwards to starting point.

Static Hold on a Gymball

The Subject should position himself in the static-hold (bridge) position on a gym ball. It is very important that the correct posture is maintained throughout the whole duration. Body must be in a straight line legs straight and together arms kept steady on the ball. Trying to hold upper body balance on the ball. Elbows must try and stays under the shoulder line maintain a 90 degree angle. The Subject must be as still and steady as possible no swinging action of the upper body Visual skills training includes total body conditioning.

Sprint forward ½ - Push-ups – Sprint forward – Push-ups – Backward Running

The Subject should sprint forward to the 10 m mark go down to complete one push-up. Explode up from push-up and sprint to the 20 m mark go down and complete another push-up. Explode up from the push-up and run backwards to the starting point. Continue this drill until the time is over.

Sprint forward ½ - Push-ups – Sprint forward – turn – Sprint forward ½ - Push-ups – Sprint forward

The Subject should sprint forward to the 10 m mark go down to complete one push-up. Explode up from push-up and sprint to the 20 m mark, touch the "line" with one hand and sprint back to the 10 m mark. Go down to the ground and complete one pushup. Explode up from the push-up and sprint to the starting point.

Sprint forward ½ x4 – Sprint forward – Push-ups – Backward running

Subject sprint forward to the 10 m mark touch the "line" with one hand and sprint back to the start – complete x4 shuttles. After completing the fourth shuttle the subject sprint to the 20 m mark. Complete one push-up and Explode up from push-up and run backwards to the starting point.

3.11.1 Description for Visual Skill Drills

Push-Up and Catch

This exercise improves the subject‟s peripheral awareness (peripheral vision), concentration and reaction time. One subject will lie down in push-up position. Stomach flat on the ground and face down (don‟t look at the thrower).On the word "**yes**" the partner must explode up from push-up position locate and catch the ball, The thrower must try and challenge the partner throw the ball wide so that the team-mate can reach for the ball make sure that the partner comes up all the way to his feet when catching the ball.

2 Vs 1

Three subjects and two cricket balls, one subject throws the ball to the "partner" to catch. When he catches the ball. He throws it back and the other subject throws a ball for the partner to catch. For the first 30 seconds the partners stands still and catch the balls. The next 30 seconds the partner shuffle one step to either side and receive the balls. The last 30 seconds is random throws. which means that the subjects can throw the balls high straight or bounce.

Simultaneous Ball Throw (SBT)

This exercise improves the subject‟s peripheral awareness (peripheral vision), concentration and ball handling skills. Bent knees, feet approximately shoulder width apart, soft hands and bring balls toward body, 1 min right hand to left hand, left hand to right hand, 1 min crossover, 1 min both balls out of hand.

Box Drill – Call

Place four beacons approximately 6 m apart in the shape of a box. Visual orientation ball drill incorporate movement drills improves the subject‟s coordination skills. Concentration and anaerobic fitness. One subject ("partner") stands at the beacon in the back right hand corner. The team-mate stands on the outside of the box and on the work "go". Team-mate calls a direction the partner must run to. E.g. if the team-mate says "forward" then the partner sprints forward and touch the beacon.

Lateral Shuffle and Ball Catch

The visual orientation ball drills incorporate movement drills. This drill improves coordination, concentration and anaerobic fitness. Place two beacons approximately 6 m apart. Subject shuffle side to side between the beacons touch the beacon on either side, look forward, head up and back kept straight, bend knees to go down or to catch the ball. Once ball is caught the subject throws it back to his team-mate. Continue shuffling side to side.

2 Vs 1 – Variation

Subjects stand in the shape of a triangle. Partner runs to his left, receives a straight ball from his team-mate. He throws the ball across to the subject standing on the right. As soon as the partner has thrown the ball he turns and runs to the other side. Receives the ball from the team-mate standing on the right side of the triangle. He throws the ball across to the subject standing on the left.

Box drill – Throw

Place 4 beacons 6 m apart (shape of a box). Partner stands in the middle of the box. Team-mate stands on the outside of the box. With two balls in his hands throw one ball anywhere in the box. Partner must catch or field the ball. Partner needs to make sure the ball doesn"t go out of the box. NB - go towards the ball, DO NOT wait for the ball is returned to the team-mate.

Crucifix Ball Drop (CBD)

Bent knees feet approximately shoulder width apart and hands on knees. Back must also be kept straight. Partner is not allowed to watch the team-mate"s hands. He must look forward when ball drops move foot quickly under ball and hand will follow – do not lunge at ball without moving feet.

Chasers

Visual orientation ball drills incorporate movement drills. This drill improves peripheral awareness, concentration and anaerobic fitness. Place 4 beacons 6 m apart and one beacon in the middle, Place a ball on a outside beacon and a ball in the middle. One subject stands in the middle and another at the outside ball. On the word "go" the subject that is in the middle takes the ball to a beacon on the outside. The outside subject takes his ball and places it on the middle beacon. He then goes and fetch the outside ball and the other subject go back to the middle beacon to fetch the ball. The aim is that the outside subject must try and catch the inside subject before he can place the ball in the middle.

Lateral Shuffle and Ball Change

Place beacons approximately 6 m apart. Tennis ball on each of the beacons and one in the middle. Partner starts in the middle with tennis ball in his hand. On the word "go" the partner shuffles sideways to a beacon BEND his knees and change the tennis balls. Shuffle then to the other side and change the balls. NB – shuffle with knees bent and on the balls of the feet.

Ladder Work with Balls

Partner stands side-on to the ladder team-mate on the opposite side of the ladder facing each other. Partner move sideways through the ladder, focus on quick feet. working on the toes, Team-mate throws cricket ball to partner while he moves through the ladder, Focus on HEAD up and eyes forward.

T-Drill

Place 3 beacons approximately 5 m apart (base). place another beacon in line with the middle beacon (in a "T" format), Subject ("partner") starts on the base at the middle beacon sprint forward; touch the top beacon with two hands in a "crouch" position, HEAD UP!, As soon as partner touch the beacon. The teammate throws the ball in any direction (left or right).Partner must try and catch the ball. Subject must try and throw the ball not to wide but must throw the ball as soon as the partner touches the beacon. Partner catches the ball with one hand, returns the ball immediately. If ball is thrown to the left then partner jogs to the left beacon on the base jog to the middle and sprint forward.

3.12 COLLECTION OF DATA – Post -test

At the end of the treatment period of twelve weeks, subjects of the two groups namely Visual Skill Fitness Training Group (VSFTG) and Control Group (CG) were tested on selected variables eye-hand co-ordination, reaction time and depth perception (visual skills variables), arm and leg explosive power, speed, agility and balance (skill related fitness variables), as such in the pre-test of the same, It was considered as post test score. The collected data were processed with appropriate statistical tool.

3.13 Statistical Technique

The following statistical procedures were employed in the present study to achieve its purposes. To test the individualized effect of both combination of VSFTG and CG on selected visual skills and skill related fitness variables, Paired t-test was used. Further, to test the comparative effects, analysis of covariance was applied. In case of significant mean difference was observed on variables used, where post-hoc test was not necessary since only two groups had been used. The level of confidence was fixed at 0.05 level.

CHAPTER IV
ANALYSIS OF DATA AND RESULTS OF THE STUDY

CHAPTER - IV

ANALYSIS AND INTERPRETATION OF DATA

In general, data may be valid, reliable and adequate but they do not serve any useful purpose unless they are carefully processed, systematically shifted, classified, tabulated, scientifically analyzed, intelligently interpreted and rationally concluded. After the data have been collected, they are analyzed using univariate and multivariate analysis. The obtained results for the individualized effect and comparative effects on variables used in the study are presented in this chapter along with a discussion on findings and hypotheses formulated for the present study.

4.1 Level of Significance

Further to test the formulated hypothesis, 0.05 level of significance is used in the study.

4.2 Result of an Individualized Effect

The results on individualized effect of Visual Skill Fitness Training Group (VSFTG) and Control Group (CG) are described in the tables of 4.1 and 4.2.

4.3 Result of t-test.

Table – 4.1

Significance of mean gains / losses between pre and post test Visual Skill Fitness training Group (VSFTG) on selected visual skills and skill related fitness variables of male cricket players

Variables	Pre test (Mean and ±S.D)	Post test (Mean and ±S.D)	MD	SE	"t"ratio
Visual Skill variables					
Eye-hand co-ordination	31.11 ±6.27	21.56 ±4.11	9.55	1.14	8.36*
Visual Reaction time	0.29 ±0.04	0.20 ±0.02	0.08	0.01	8.92*
Depth perception	3.79 ±1.91	2.43 ±1.28	1.37	0.27	5.00*
Skill Related Fitness Variables					
Arm explosive power	4.01 ±0.45	4.49 ±0.35	0.48	0.06	7.88*
Leg explosive power	47.60 ±3.36	58.33 ±3.56	10.73	0.73	14.77*
Speed	7.43 ±0.39	6.68 ±0.39	0.75	0.08	8.89*
Agility	18.02 ±0.65	16.10 ±0.62	1.92	0.15	13.09*
Balance	21.80 ±3.85	33.93 ±5.26	12.13	0.90	13.50*

*Significant at 0.05 level: 2.14

Table 4.1 indicates that the obtained „t" values of the visual skill fitness training group (VSFTG) on variables are: 8.36 (eye-hand co-ordination) 8.92 (visual reaction time), 5.00 (depth perception), 7.88 (arm explosive power), 14.77 (leg explosive power), 8.89 (speed), 13.09 (agility) and 13.50 (balance). The obtained t- values are significant at 0.05 levels for degree of freedom 1, 14 and the required critical value is 2.14. Hence the obtained t-values on the selected variables are higher than the required critical value, it is concluded that the visual skill fitness training group, has produced significant changes positively from its baseline to post treatment on selected visual skills and skill related fitness variables of eye hand coordination (+9.55 $P<0.05$), visual reaction time (+0.08$P<0.05$), depth perception (+1.37$P<0.05$) arm explosive power (+0.48$P<0.05$), leg explosive power (+10.73$P<0.05$), speed (+0.75$P<0.05$), agility (+1.92$P<0.05$), and balance (+12.13$P<0.05$).

The changes made from the baseline to the post treatment of Visual Skill Fitness Training Group (VSFTG) on selected visual skills variables (eye-hand co-ordination, visual reaction time and depth perception) and skill related fitness (arm explosive power and leg explosive power, speed, agility and balance) were displayed in Figures 4.1 to Figures 4.8.

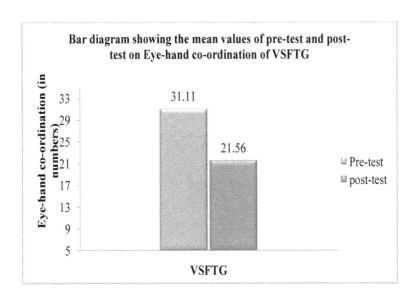

Fig – 4.1

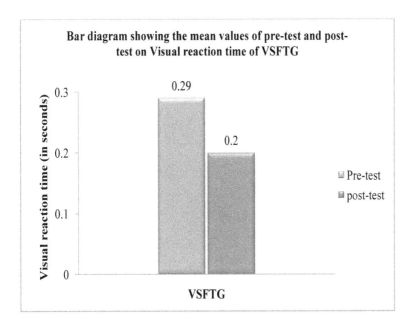

Fig – 4.2

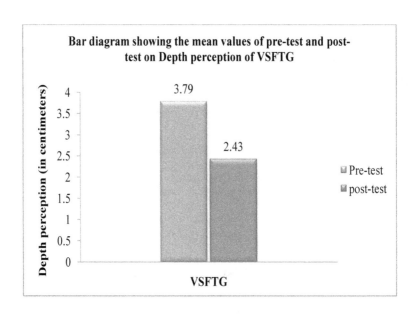

Fig – 4.3

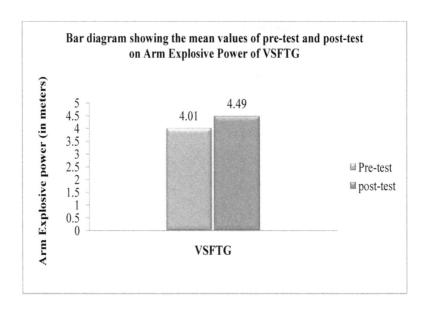

Fig – 4.4

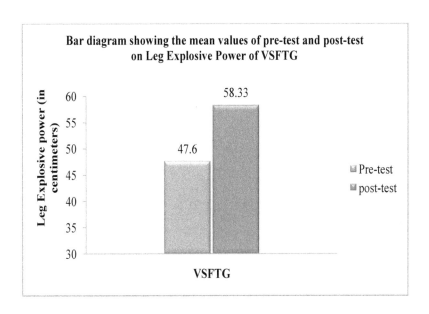

Fig – 4.5

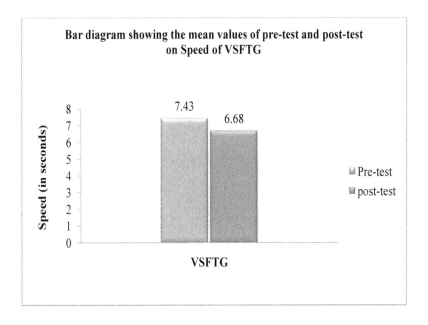

Fig – 4.6

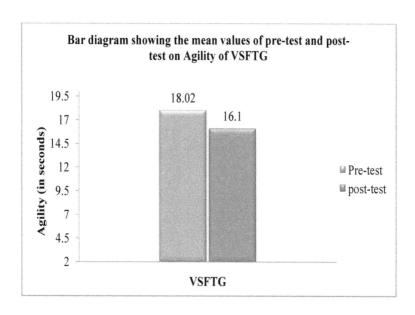

Fig – 4.7

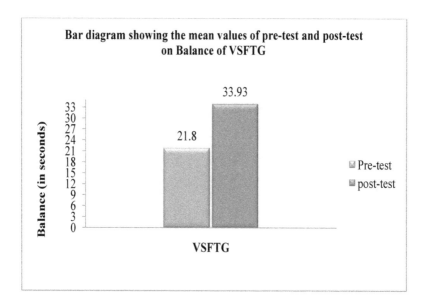

Fig – 4.8

Table – 4.2

Significance of mean gains / losses between pre and post test Control Group (CG) on on selected visual skills and skill related fitness variables of male cricket players

Variables	Pre test (Mean and ±S.D)	Post test (Mean and ±S.D)	MD	SE	„t"ratio
Visual Skill variables					
Eye-hand co-ordination	29.29 ±12.46	28.46 ±11.66	0.83	0.43	1.93
Visual Reaction time	0.27 ±0.03	0.28 ±0.03	0.02	0.01	1.75
Depth perception	3.40 ±1.03	3.29 ±0.86	0.11	0.07	1.65
Skill Related Fitness Variables					
Arm explosive power	3.84 ±0.50	3.95 ±0.49	0.11	0.04	3.19*
Leg explosive power	47.73 ±4.74	49.87 ±4.69	2.13	0.24	9.03*
Speed	7.30 ±0.47	7.06 ±0.35	0.24	0.08	2.86*
Agility	18.29 ±0.57	18.13 ±0.42	0.16	0.09	1.77
Balance	19.07 ±3.63	20.60 ±3.29	1.53	0.19	7.99*

*Significant at 0.05 level: 2.14

Table 4.2 indicates that the obtained „t"values of the control group (CG) on variables are: 1.93 (eye-hand co-ordination), 1.75 (visual reaction time), 1.65 (depth perception) and 1.77 (agility). The obtained t- values are significant at 0.05 levels for degree of freedom 1, 14 and the required critical value is 2.14. Hence the obtained t-values on the variables were failed to reach the significant level. It was concluded that the changes made from pre-test to post test was statistically not significant.

The obtained „t"values of the control group (CG) on variables are: 3.19 (arm explosive power), 9.03 (leg explosive power), 2.86 (speed) and 7.99 (balance). The obtained t- values are significant at 0.05 levels for degree of freedom 1, 14 and the required critical value is 2.14. Hence the obtained t-values on the selected variables are higher than the required critical value, it is concluded that the control group, has produced significant changes positively from its baseline to post treatment on selected skill related fitness variables of arm explosive power (+0.11P<0.05), leg explosive power (+2.13P<0.05), speed (+0.24P<0.05) and balance (+1.53P<0.05).

The changes made from the baseline to the post treatment of Control Group (CG) on selected visual skills variables (eye-hand co-ordination, visual reaction time and depth perception) and skill related fitness (arm explosive power and leg explosive power, speed, agility and balance) were displayed in Figures 4.9 to Figures 4.16.

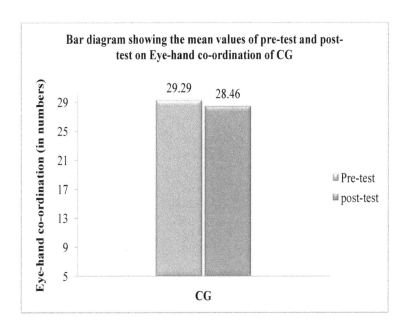

Fig – 4.9

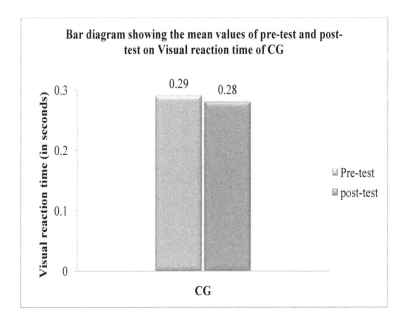

Fig – 4.10

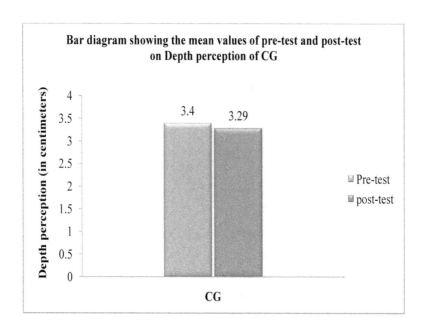

Fig – 4.11

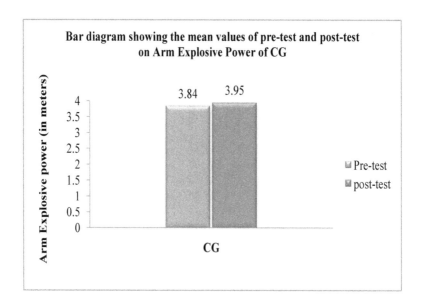

Fig – 4.12

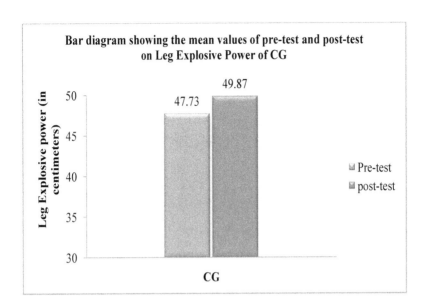

Fig – 4.13

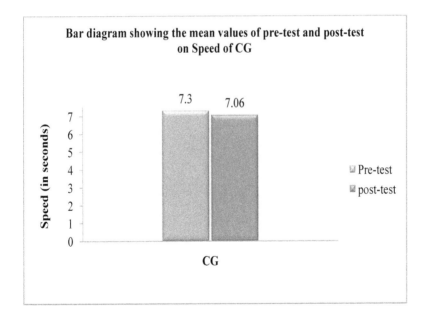

Fig – 4.14

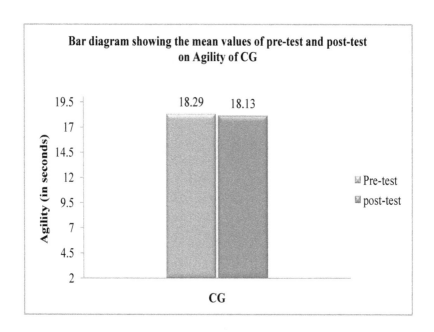

Fig – 4.15

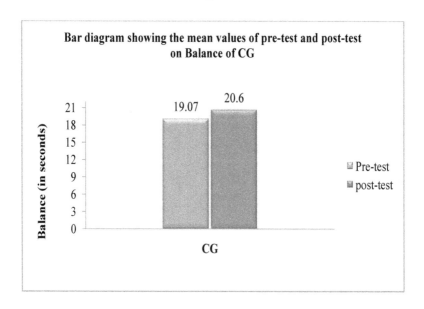

Fig – 4.16

4.4 Result of Analysis of Variance.

Table 4.3 showing the computation of analysis of variance of initial and final means on selected visual skills and skill related fitness variables namely eye-hand co-ordination, visual reaction time, depth perception arm explosive power, leg explosive power, speed, agility and balance.

Table - 4.3
Computation of Analysis of Variance of Initial means of Visual skills and skill related fitness variables

Variables	Sources	SS	DF	MS	F-ratio
Eye –hand coordination	Between sets	24.90	1	24.90	0.25
	Within sets	2761.01	28	98.61	
Visual reaction time	Between sets	0.00	1	0.00	0.38
	Within sets	0.03	28	0.00	
Depth perception	Between sets	1.14	1	1.14	0.46
	Within sets	69.46	28	2.48	
Arm explosive power	Between sets	0.22	1	0.22	0.94
	Within sets	6.54	28	0.23	
Leg explosive power	Between sets	0.13	1	0.13	0.01
	Within sets	472.53	28	16.88	
Speed	Between sets	0.12	1	0.12	0.61
	Within sets	5.38	28	0.19	
Agility	Between sets	0.59	1	0.59	1.50
	Within sets	10.97	28	0.39	
Balance	Between sets	56.03	1	56.03	3.85
	Within sets	407.33	28	14.55	

*significant at 0.05 level

Table - 4.4

Computation of Analysis of Variance of Final means of Visual skills and skill related fitness variables

Eye –hand coordination	Between sets	356.94	1	356.94	4.63*
	Within sets	2157.27	28	77.05	
Visual reaction time	Between sets	0.04	1	0.04	51.21*
	Within sets	0.02	28	0.00	
Depth perception	Between sets	5.62	1	5.62	4.51*
	Within sets	34.87	28	1.25	
Arm explosive power	Between sets	2.14	1	2.14	11.49*
	Within sets	5.21	28	0.19	
Leg explosive power	Between sets	537.63	1	537.63	31.03*
	Within sets	485.07	28	17.32	
Speed	Between sets	1.08	1	1.08	7.49*
	Within sets	4.03	28	0.14	
Agility	Between sets	31.07	1	31.07	106.80*
	Within sets	8.15	28	0.29	
Balance	Between sets	1333.33	1	1333.33	65.90*
	Within sets	566.53	28	20.23	

*significant at 0.05 level

4.5. Results on Testing the Initials and Final Means

In the initial data analysis, F-test was applied to test initial and final means between the group of Visual Skill Fitness Training Group (VSFTG) and Control Group (CG) on selected visual skill and skill related fitness variables such as eye-hand co-ordination, visual reaction time, depth perception, arm explosive power, leg explosive power, speed, agility, and balance. The F-value needed for significance for DF 1, 28 is at 0.05 levels is 4.21.

The obtained F-value (table 4.3) for the initial means on selected visual skill and skill related fitness variables are 0.25 (eye – hand co-ordination), 0.38 (visual reaction time), 0.46 (depth perception), 0.94 (arm explosive power), 0.01 (leg explosive power), 0.61 (speed), 1.50 (agility) and 3.85 (balance). Since the obtained critical value failed to reach the required critical value 4.21 for df 1, 28, it was found to be insignificant. It is concluded that the mean difference between the VSFTG and CG on the variables used in this study before the treatment (Figs 4.1 to 4.8) is statistically non significant.

The observed F-Value (table 4.4) for the final means are 4.63 (eye –hand co-ordination), 51.21 (visual reaction time), 4.51 (depth perception), 11.49 (arm explosive power), 31.03 (leg explosive power), 7.49 (speed), 106.80 (agility) and 65.90 (balance). These values are compared to the critical value at significant level, and it is found that the observed F-Values on final means of eye-hand co-ordination, visual reaction time, depth perception, arm explosive power, leg explosive power, speed, agility and balance are greater than the significant level. Therefore it is concluded that the mean difference between the VSFTG and CG on final means of the variables are statistically significant.

4.6 Results of Analysis of Covariance

Table 4.5 to Table 4.12 showing the computation of analysis of covariance on variable namely eye-hand co-ordination, visual reaction time, depth perception, arm explosive power, leg explosive power, speed, agility and balance.

Table – 4.5
Analysis of Covariance of Adjusted Post test means on Eye-hand coordination

VSFTG	CG	Sources	SS	DF	MS	F-ratio
20.8	29.22	Between sets	526.77	1	526.77	60.06*
		Within sets	236.82	27	8.77	

*significant at 0.05 level

The table 4.5 reveals that adjusted post test means values on VFSTG (20.80) and CG (29.22). The obtained „f" value was 60.06. To be significant at 0.05 level for degree of freedom 1, 27, the required critical value was 4.21. Hence, observed „f" value (60.06) was found as higher than the table value (4.21), it was inferred that the adjusted mean difference existing between the VSFTG and CG on eye-hand co-ordination was statistically significant.

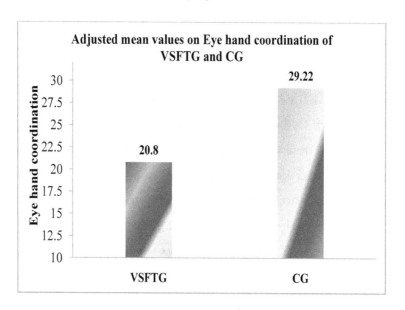

Fig – 4.17

Table – 4.6

Analysis of Covariance of Adjusted Post test means on Visual reaction time

VSFTG	CG	Sources	SS	DF	MS	F-ratio
0.20	0.28	Between sets	0.04	1	0.04	50.26*
		Within sets	0.02	27	0.00	

*significant at 0.05 level

The table 4.6 reveals that adjusted post test means values on VFSTG (0.20) and CG (0.28). The obtained „f"value was 50.26. To be significant at 0.05 level for degree of freedom 1, 27, the required critical value was 4.21. Hence, observed „f"value (50.26) was found as higher than the table value (4.21), it was inferred that the adjusted mean difference existing between the VSFTG and CG on visual reaction time was statistically significant.

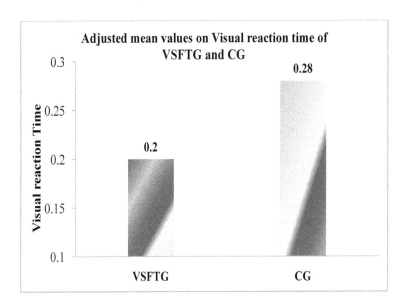

Fig – 4.18

Table – 4.7

Analysis of Covariance of Adjusted Post test means on Depth perception

VSFTG	CG	Sources	SS	DF	MS	F-ratio
2.30	3.42	Between sets	9.13	1	9.13	34.50*
		Within sets	7.14	27	0.26	

*significant at 0.05 level

The table 4.7 reveals that adjusted post test means values on VFSTG (2.30) and CG (3.42). The obtained „f"value was 34.50. To be significant at 0.05 level for degree of freedom 1, 27, the required critical value was 4.21. Hence, observed „f"value (34.50) was found as higher than the table value (4.21), it was inferred that the adjusted mean difference existing between the VSFTG and CG on depth perception was statistically significant.

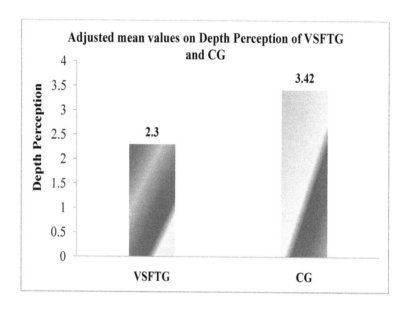

Fig – 4.19

Table – 4.8

Analysis of Covariance of Adjusted Post test means on Arm explosive power

VSFTG	CG	Sources	SS	DF	MS	F-ratio
4.42	4.02	Between sets	1.13	1	1.13	36.41*
		Within sets	0.83	27	0.03	

*significant at 0.05 level

The table 4.8 reveals that adjusted post test means values on VFSTG (4.42) and CG (4.02). The obtained „f"value was 36.41. To be significant at 0.05 level for degree of freedom 1, 27, the required critical value was 4.21. Hence, observed „f"value (36.41) was found as higher than the table value (4.21), it was inferred that the adjusted mean difference existing between the VSFTG and CG on arm explosive power was statistically significant.

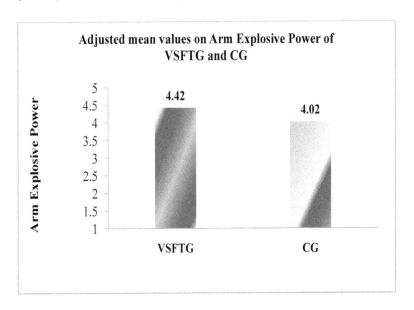

Fig – 4.20

Table – 4.9

Analysis of Covariance of Adjusted Post test means on Leg explosive power

VSFTG	CG	Sources	SS	DF	MS	F-ratio
58.39	49.81	Between sets	552.54	1	552.54	128.33*
		Within sets	116.25	27	4.31	

*significant at 0.05 level

The table 4.9 reveals that adjusted post test means values on VFSTG (58.39) and CG (49.81). The obtained „f"value was 128.33. To be significant at 0.05 level for degree of freedom 1, 27, the required critical value was 4.21. Hence, observed „f"value (128.33) was found as higher than the table value (4.21), it was inferred that the adjusted mean difference existing between the VSFTG and CG on leg explosive power was statistically significant.

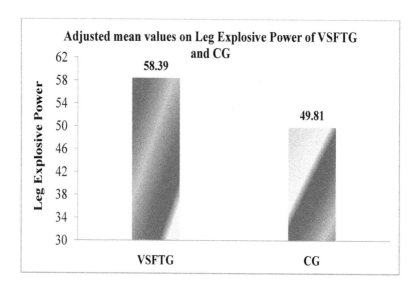

Fig – 4.21

Table – 4.10

Analysis of Covariance of Adjusted Post test means on Speed

VSFTG	CG	Sources	SS	DF	MS	F-ratio
6.64	7.10	Between sets	1.51	1	1.51	19.37*
		Within sets	2.11	27	0.08	

*significant at 0.05 level

The table 4.10 reveals that adjusted post test means values on VFSTG (6.64) and CG (7.10). The obtained „f"value was 19.37. To be significant at 0.05 level for degree of freedom 1, 27, the required critical value was 4.21. Hence, observed „f" value (19.37) was found as higher than the table value (4.21), it was inferred that the adjusted mean difference existing between the VSFTG and CG on speed was statistically significant.

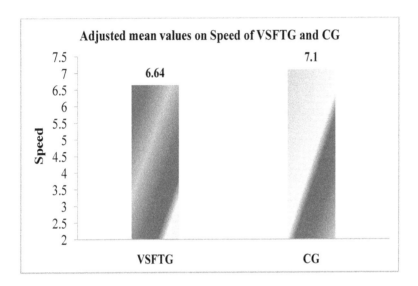

Fig – 4.22

Table – 4.11

Analysis of Covariance of Adjusted Post test means on Agility

VSFTG	CG	Sources	SS	DF	MS	F-ratio
16.18	18.05	Between sets	24.93	1	24.93	153.25*
		Within sets	4.39	27	0.16	

*significant at 0.05 level

The table 4.11 reveals that adjusted post test means values on VFSTG (16.18) and CG (18.05). The obtained „f"value was 153.25. To be significant at 0.05 level for degree of freedom 1, 27, the required critical value was 4.21. Hence, observed „f"value (153.25) was found as higher than the table value (4.21), it was inferred that the adjusted mean difference existing between the VSFTG and CG on agility was statistically significant.

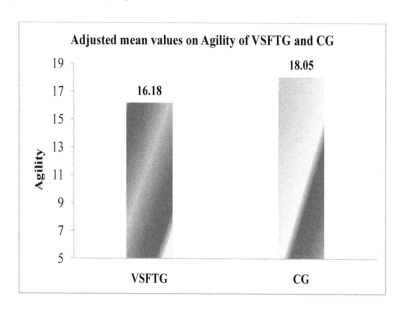

Fig – 4.23

Table – 4.12

Analysis of Covariance of Adjusted Post test means on Balance

VSFTG	CG	Sources	SS	DF	MS	F-ratio
32.60	21.94	Between sets	749.39	1	749.39	114.14*
		Within sets	177.26	27	6.57	

*significant at 0.05 level

The table 4.12 reveals that adjusted post test means values on VFSTG (32.60) and CG (21.94). The obtained „f" value was 114.14. To be significant at 0.05 level for degree of freedom 1, 27, the required critical value was 4.21. Hence, observed „f" value (114.14) was found as higher than the table value (4.21), it was inferred that the adjusted mean difference existing between the VSFTG and CG on balance was statistically significant.

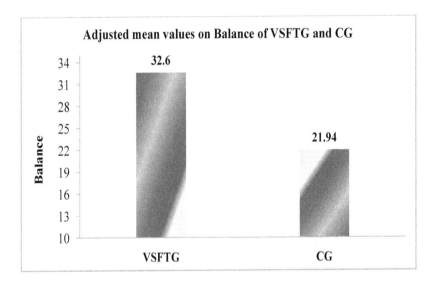

Fig – 4.24

4.7 Discussion on Findings

Cricket is a team game involves the fundamental skills of fielding, bowling, batting and catching. In India, the game cricket is a very popular game among the peoples even in the tiny villages as the game is not financially constraint and seemed to be a recreate cum competitive in nature. In international sport arena specifically in the game of cricket in India made remarkable contributions in terms of achievements. With such interest, students in schools and colleges are highly motivating themselves to participate and to become an outstanding players in future. As for as their learning in fundamental skills, one can confidently assures that the prime sources might be of their self learning they have been through television or seeing matches directly. Following this, when they go for training and coaching, their system is an emphasis mostly physical and motor aspect even this game is highly demanded by the coordinative abilities which are required in bowling and catching the ball besides batting. Coordinative abilities include visual skills such as reaction, perception, and balance. Mastering in the coordinative abilities helps the player to execute the fundamental skills successfully. In this regard the appropriate means are visual skill fitness training program. Visual skills fitness training exercises allows sportsmen to improve their visual skills as well as improve their performance skills. Thus it helps to the players to perform at their best and helping the players to reach the next level visual skills fitness training is becoming more essential as it ensures optimal performance of elite cricket players. With being sport is big business globally, everybody involved to recognize the essential need to develop their visual and mental abilities rather than training physical abilities and skills to achieve that edge over the competitors.

With this aim, the present study was conducted to find out the effect of visual skill fitness training programme on selected visual skill and skill related fitness variables of male cricket players. The collected data on this treated with analysis of covariance as to compare the effects of visual skill fitness training with the traditional training program to the development of visual skill and skill related fitness variables. The derived results of analysis of co-variance on comparative effects between the groups of VSFTG and CG on selected visual skills and skill related fitness variables, explained that the subjects are treated with VSFTG have performed, better in visual skills (eye-hand co-ordination, visual reaction time, depth perception) and skill related fitness (arm explosive power, leg explosive power, speed, agility, balance) are compared to players treated with CG only. Therefore, the visual skill fitness training group performed superior in the selected visual skills and skill related fitness performance variables of male cricket players, than the players practiced with conventional training alone. The sources for the dominance of VSFTG over to CG on variables used in the study are discussed with the research studies and theories related to this as follows.

In analyze the results on visual skills namely, eye hand coordination, visual reaction time and balance, the observed results are favored to players practiced with the specifically designed program of visual skill fitness training. Visual skills training exercises, like any other component of the player"s training regime, are necessary for optimal preparation for competition and can be used as specialized training which involves improving the peak visual skills for the cricketers, such as following a ball, to be able to react more quickly, judging depth accurately and hand eye co-ordination.

Eye hand coordination plays an important role in the cricket because of coordination is a needed factors for any skills in the game. During the bowling time in each and every ball movement, players mind would focus on the bowlers" action. At the same time he wants to face that ball with hand and foot coordination. Sometimes players using only footwork, at the same time want to use eye- hand coordination also, otherwise can"t able to meet the ball in a right direction. Regarding the visual skill of balance in cricket, players have to play for a long time in the field, they wants to be balance the body for the entire situation while facing the ball and receiving the ball in fielding position. The visual skill fitness training players using ball drop, alternate catch drill and push-ups and catch. These drills are improving the balance performance. In addition to this, the ball movement in this game is not only so short and also very long in nature. Players should have the ability to perceive the ball in the right distance at right time which enables them to execute their skills successfully. Mastering these skills indirectly helps to the subjects for their development visual reaction time. For which they have to perform better in depth perception. Having the nature of these skills the VSFT program was designed so as to develop the visual skills

In the visual skill fitness training drills used as exercises are mostly related to the skills in the game of cricket. Visual skills training exercises is a method of performance to enhancement that has been proven to take the players at all the levels of competition to the next level, the drills that were used in this study is totally safe as well as completely legal, and it has only positive consequences both on and off the field. Vision training consists of a variety of programmes to enhance the player"s visual performance. Wood and Abernethy (1997) stated that vision training was consists of a variety of programmes to enhance visual performance.

The visual system plays a crucial role in guiding the player"s search for essential information underlying skilful behavior. The process of selecting relevant information, whilst disregarding the less informative pieces of information is not conducted in an arbitrary manner. It is based on the deliberate visual search strategies (Bard & Fleury, 1976). It has been argued that visual skills training exercises allow athletes to improve their visual skills and also improve their performance skills. Wilson and Falkel (2004) stated that the improvements from visual skills training exercises in eye movement skills, focusing skills, peripheral visual awareness, and visual perceptual skills can carry over onto the field of play. According to Abernethy (1996) the role of vision can generally be accepted as a critical source of information for the planning and the executing of motor skills. Planer (1994) reported that eye-hand-body coordination and visual adjustability are interdependent of each other. The latter is concerned with the ability of the body to adjust various motor movements quickly, as a reaction to a stimulus, where the stimulus is the ability of the eyes to integrate with the body as a unit.

Vision is the ability to process or interpret the information which is seen Loran (1995). Previously, vision training and visual skills were not considered to be that important in the everyday sport setting, although athletes and trainers did do vision related training tests inadvertently. Research has now shown that the importance of visual skills is based on the performance of an athlete (Miyao M., 1993, Rouse et al., 1989, Williams, 1975 and Christenson, 1988). Williams and Grant (1999) explained that hand-eye co-ordination involves the integration of the eyes and the hands/body as a unit. Thus the eyes must lead and guide the motor system of the body (also known as the movement system). When a deficit is found in hand-eye co-ordination, it can be expected that the deficit can have an effect of all levels of performance that require movement of the player, bat, ball, etc. Since, sport is typically performed under temporal constraints and varying levels of physiological stress or fatigue, attempts should be made to examine visual function under more realistic test conditions. Planer (1994) explained that the quick identification of objects as they move through space rely on aspects of eye movements, focus flexibility, fusion flexibility and depth perception. The author explained that these relates to the ability of the eyes to work together when watching and moving object, to quickly with simultaneously change focus with minimum effort, to fuse these objects together, and then to use these clear fused images quickly so as to perceive depth.

Thus the scientific nature of visual skill fitness training might have been the source for the dominance of VSFT group on eye hand coordination, balance, depth perception and visual reaction time compared to the subjects of control group. Findings on the visual skills are substantiated by the following research studies. From the findings of Wilson and Falkel (2004) has stated that visual skills plays a very important role in that specific activity as they significantly affect batting averages in cricket. These studies relied on empirical data from a vision training group and a control group given no vision training. These studies claimed to show the benefits of visual skills training in improving static balance and hand-eye coordination (McLeod & Hansen, 1989b; McLeod, 1991). According to Lee (1980) "if play encourages normal gross motor development and improves eye-hand and eye-body co-ordination with peripheral vision helps to develop these basic motor skills, it has then clear that vision and motor skills are linked to sports performance".

Following this, the results on fitness variables of arm explosive power, leg explosive power speed, and agility also the subjects of VSFT were found to be higher in the performance as compared to the subjects of conventional training group. The source for such a significant result produced on fitness variables may be because of the salient feature of VSFT used in this study. In VSFT practice the fielding drills they want to be collect the ball, then after collecting the ball and throw to their target point. In this drill arm explosive power playing major role, in visual skill fitness training players practicing medicine ball throw with different weights according to their capability. In visual skills fitness training they using running drills forward sprint, backward running and push-ups for improving their skill related fitness performance. In visual skill drills players doing all skill related drills like push-up and catch and partner catch etc.

Regarding running drills and visual skill related drills twenty meter distance to be fixed for all the running drills. In running drills mainly they are doing shuttle run, forward sprint, backward running, ladder run, push-ups, medicine ball throw, and pushups and hold etc., the intensity of the training was fixed gradually increased for all the three phases. In visual skill drills push-ups and catch, partner catch, ladder run and catch, ball drop and catch, lateral shuffle and receiving the ball on alternate side etc., So that visual skill fitness training programme improves visual skills as well as skill related physical fitness variables (arm explosive power, leg explosive power, speed, and agility). Besides physical fitness variables are discussed briefly as follows. As for as arm explosive power and leg explosive power are concerned both are essential fitness components in the game of cricket. The game of cricket practically arm explosive power was very essential in fielding, batting and bowling. When the players hitting the ball hardly means at that time arm power is needed, in fielding players want to be field the ball and throw the ball in their correct target point, in bowling players using more power to releasing the ball. Leg explosive power is an essential in bowling action specifically during the bowler"s takeoff and catching the ball in the boundary line for high catches. In bowling action bowler gradually increasing their speed and finally before releasing the ball bowler want to take off with lifting her leg high level. With this thrust the drills were designed in the VSFT. In the VSFT in running drills medicine ball throw also concerned one of the drills. Medicine ball forward and backward throw were used for all the subjects. Players practicing their regular medicine ball practices for two days a week over a period of twelve weeks. So that arm explosive power was increased. In running and visual skill drills all the players involving in ladder jumping movements.

When discussing the sources for VSFT dominance over the fitness variable of speed and agility was gradual increase of training load in all the three phases in the running drills and visual skill drills players are also doing all the skills in short distance. Speed is an important component for all the game. Especially in cricket batting and bowling plays very important role. In running between the wickets speed also include. After hitting the ball players want to reach the opponent grease before opponent throwing to the target point. In some times players started the run but partner gave the call no, so that players want to return the grease as soon possible otherwise he will lose the wicket. In bowling bowlers are gradually increasing the speed to releasing the ball with maximum speed. The visual skills and skill related drills players doing their movements in various directions. For example, chasers, box drill and lateral shuffle and ball change etc. these drills improving the agility performance. In practical game players can change the body movements according to their ball direction and to stop the ball. For each and every ball the players must keeps her body movement ready to receiving the ball for all the situations.

CHAPTER V
SUMMARY, CONCLUSIONS AND RECOMMENDATIONS

CHAPTER - V
SUMMARY, CONCLUSION AND RECOMMENDATION

5.1 Summary

In the game of cricket effectiveness of the player's ability to act quickly and accurately depends upon how efficient the visual system can process the information. Visual information is critical for performing a variety of motor skills that are used in cricket. When the players' movements must coincide with a changing environment, such as hitting the ball, catching the ball, or in motor activities requiring precise movements of the limbs in regards to a target. Having this the present study was formed with the thirst of finding the changes on visual skills fitness variables when imparting the visual skill fitness training in addition to their physical training schedule in the game of cricket. The present study has been carried with the title "Effects of visual skills fitness training programme on selected on visual skills and skill related fitness variables of male cricket players".

To achieve the purpose of the study, male cricket players were selected as samples (N=134) who were the participants of inter-collegiate level cricket tournament. Their overall playing ability was measured using ten point rating scale by three experts in the game of cricket. Being the player, and coach, investigator was also one among them in measuring the overall playing ability. The performance of a player in the game was considered as overall playing ability. Based on their performance those who scored in the range of 4 to 5 were considered for further study. Thus the samples selected were 52. From them 30 players were selected randomly as subjects for this present study. In present study as experiment design, pre-post random experiment group design was applied to study the effect of visual skills training. For this, the subjects selected (N=30), were assigned randomly into two groups namely experimental group and control group. The experimental group-1 was named as Visual Skills Fitness Training Group (VSFTG), and Control Group (CG). In the present study the subjects used for control group were practiced with their own training schedule. Each group was consisting of 15 subjects. The subjects selected for this study were hailed from various socio-economic conditions. Their age was fixed in the range of 19 – 24 years.

The subjects of two groups were measured on the following variables: eye-hand coordination, visual reaction time and depth perception (visual skills), arm explosive power, leg explosive power, speed, agility and balance (skill related fitness). Thus the collected data were considered as pre-test score for the present study. After completion of pre test, the players of Visual Skill Fitness Training Group (VSFTG) underwent visual skill fitness training programme for two days a week for about twelve weeks in addition to their traditional training. Subjects in the control group were not engaged in any specific training perform other than traditional way of practice activity practice during the training period. After the completion of twelve weeks of treatment period, the subjects of VSFTG and CG were tested on selected visual skills and skill related fitness variables as such in the case of pre test. It was considered as post test score.

The collected data were processed with paired t – test to study the individualized effects, so as to study the changes from pre-test to post test on selected visual skills and skill related variables. Further, analysis of covariance was used to study the comparative effects between the visual skill fitness training group and control group on selected visual skills and skill related fitness variables of male inter collegiate cricket players. The level of significance chosen to test the derived results was 0.05 which considered being appropriate for this study.

5.2 Results

In testing the individualized effect of visual skill fitness training and control group, the results observed are as follows.

1. In studying the changes observed from, base line to post treatment of visual skill fitness training, significant changes have been observed positively on selected visual skills (eye-hand coordination, visual reaction time and depth perception) and skill related fitness variables (speed, agility, arm explosive power, leg explosive power and balance). Further, in studying the changes observed from the baseline to the post treatment on subjects of control group, significant changes was observed on selected visual skill related fitness variables such as speed, arm explosive power and leg explosive power and balance) whereas in the case of agility and visual skills no significant changes was observed.

2. In testing the comparative effects of visual skill fitness training and control group, the obtained results are positively favored to the VSFT on selected visual skills (eye-hand coordination, visual reaction time and depth perception) and skill related fitness variables of arm explosive power and leg explosive power, speed, agility and balance when compared to players pertain to control group.

5.3 Conclusions

Based on the results the following conclusions have been made.

In visual skills of eye-hand coordination, visual reaction time and depth perception, the subjects of VSFT were significantly performed better as compared to players practiced with conventional training (control group). Based on the results, it was concluded that the combined effect of visual skills and running drills used to develop the fitness related parameters and skill related parameters might have been the source for dominance over the visual skills variables when compared to control group.

Further in the case of skill related fitness aspects such as arm explosive power, leg explosive power, speed, agility and balance, the derived results favored to the subjects of VSFT compared to the players practiced with conventional training. In examine the significant effect of VSFT over the dominance on skill related fitness variables compared to control group, it was concluded that exercises designed specifically for this underlie the medicine ball throw and strength and power related drills to develop visual skills, may be the significant sources.

5.4   Recommendations

1. Many aspects of the cricket player"s abilities can be greatly enhanced by cricket specific training drills, the player"s visual perceptual and visual motor abilities can be dramatically improved by introducing visual skills fitness training programmes.

2. The training sessions should be engaging and appropriate to cricket. By using cricket specific vision enhancement activities on the field, it will enable the coach and the player to see remarkable improvements in overall performance.

3. For a coach to gain the most out of the training sessions, it is recommended that the coach highlight the key visual information used during practice sessions and by doing this it might lead to more effective performance.

4. In planning daily practices, these visual perceptual skill exercises that were used for the purpose of this study can easily be incorporated into regular practice activities.

5. Vision training is a new concept, which is like strength training where specific visual skills can be improved by isolating and training them separately. This is especially rewarding when athletes' performance reaches its threshold and further enhancement could be achieved by vision training.

CPSIA information can be obtained
at www.ICGtesting.com
Printed in the USA
LVHW050104260123
737950LV00015B/1254